"This book is long overdue. Its PRACTICAL, 'HANDS ON' APPROACH to treating chemically dependent people with HIV illness is of invaluable help to those working with this population. What shines through these chapters is the courage and spirit of both those afflicted by chemical dependency and HIV illness and those who care for them."

—Emily B. McNally, PhD, CAC, Co-Author, *Dual Identities: Counseling Chemically Dependent Gay Men & Lesbians;*
Co-Director, Discovery Counseling Center, New York City

"A remarkable and extraordinarily helpful book on work with HIV-infected drug users. Any reader beginning work with such clients will find valuable information and guidance from any chapter in the book, and experienced practitioners will both broaden and deepen their store of knowledge and enrich their work by use of various chapters. The author's use of case examples concretizes their points and gives the reader a realistic sense of what work is like with this client population. Certainly, the number of practitioners counseling chemically dependent clients with HIV will increase as the number of such clients continues to grow. THE SOCIAL WORK AND COUNSELING PROFESSIONS NEED THIS BOOK NOW."

—Ralph J. Burant, Editor, *Families in Society*

Counseling Chemically Dependent People with HIV Illness

Counseling Chemically Dependent People with HIV Illness

Michael Shernoff
Editor

Counseling Chemically Dependent People with HIV Illness, edited by Michael Shernoff, was simultaneously issued by The Haworth Press, Inc., under the same title, as special issue of the *Journal of Chemical Dependency Treatment*, Volume 4, Number 2, 1991, Dana Finnegan, Editor.

Harrington Park Press
An Imprint of The Haworth Press, Inc.
New York • London

ISBN 1-56023-016-9

Published by

Harrington Park Press, 10 Alice Street, Binghamton, NY 13904-1580

Harrington Park Press is an imprint of The Haworth Press, Inc., 10 Alice Street, Binghamton, NY 13904-1580.

Counseling Chemically Dependent People with HIV Illness was originally published as *Journal of Chemical Dependency Treatment*, Volume 4, Number 2 1991.

Library of Congress Cataloging-in-Publication Data

Counseling chemically dependent people with HIV illness / Michael Shernoff, editor.
    p. cm.
    Simultaneously issued by Haworth Press under the same title, as a special issue of the journal of chemical dependency treatment, v. 4, no. 2, 1991.
    ISBN 1-56023-016-9 (HPP : alk. paper)
    1. Substance abuse – Patients – Counseling of. 2. HIV infections – Patients – Counseling of. 3. HIV infections – Patients – Substance use. 4. AIDS (Disease) – Patients – Counseling of. 5. AIDS (Disease) – Patients – Substance use. I. Shernoff, Michael, 1951- .
    [DNLM: 1. Counseling – methods. 2. HIV infections. 3. Substance Dependence. WM 55 C8533]
RC564.C694 1991b
616.86'0651 – dc20
DNLM/DLC   91-35376
for Library of Congress   CIP

Dedication

To the memory of Luis Palacios-Jiminez, CSW, ACSW,
(December 6, 1952 – June 13, 1989)
social worker, psychotherapist, AIDS educator,
colleague and friend . . .
another casualty of AIDS.

ABOUT THE EDITOR

Michael Shernoff, CSW, ACSW, is founder and co-director of Chelsea Psychotherapy Associates in Manhattan. He is adjunct faculty at Hunter College Graduate School of Social Work and is a board member of The National Lesbian/Gay Health Foundation. He has co-chaired the AIDS Task Force for both the Society for the Scientific Study of Sex and The American Orthopsychiatric Association. He co-edited The Sourcebook on Lesbian/Gay Health Care, Volumes 1 and 2 and is co-author of three of the most widely used AIDS prevention interventions for gay and bisexual men in the world. He co-authored The Facilitator's Guide to Eroticizing Safer Sex and numerous articles on AIDS prevention and mental health issues pertaining to lesbians and gay men. He lectures on these issues around the United States.

CONTENTS

Introduction

Michael Shernoff, MSW

In early 1982 I was hired as the Counseling Supervisor at Greenwich House West Methadone Maintenance Treatment Program located in Manhattan's Chelsea neighborhood. There I had the good fortune to meet Dr. Lawrence Mass, who was medical director of this agency. I was already familiar with Dr. Mass through his writings in the New York Native about a devastating new disease that was affecting gay men. It was a privilege to become colleagues with this brilliant, visionary, and caring physician, who had the courage to continue to attempt to alert both the general public and medical profession about a newly emerging public health disaster.

It was Dr. Mass who first brought to my attention that some of the patients we were treating at the methadone program were having abnormal blood chemistries and were beginning to suffer from unusual illnesses not often seen, even in poor, malnourished drug-addicted individuals. Dr. Mass made it a point to share his medical observations with the entire staff during our case review meetings. This was the first inclination I had that something was medically amiss in a new way with people who had a history of using drugs intravenously. It wasn't until several months later that Dr. Mass and others began to connect what was occurring to gay men with what they were observing in people who had a history of I.V. drug use.

Now, ten years later it is common knowledge that AIDS is devastating several communities of people. Since the vast majority of people who have gotten AIDS through I.V. drug use are poor and people of color, the organized governmental response to meeting their medical and psycho-social needs has been even more abysmal than the minimum response extorted from the health care system

1

and government by middle class gay men. Even today there are drug treatment professionals and centers that try not to work with people who are infected with HIV or who have AIDS.

Though some articles began appearing in the professional literature as early as 1984 (Marmor, DesJarlais et al, 1984), it was not until Dr. Larry Siegel edited a ground breaking book on AIDS and substance abuse in 1988 that the issues inherent in working with this population impacted by AIDS began to be addressed in depth. This current volume is entirely different from Dr. Siegel's pioneering and important work. I have invited several men and women who are on the front lines of treating chemically dependent individuals who are infected with HIV or who have full-blown AIDS to share what it is exactly that they are doing while working with this very difficult client population. My goal in conceiving of this book was that when other professionals in the field of chemical dependency read the chapters in this volume they will gain a better understanding of how to work with their own chemically dependent clients who have HIV illness more effectively. Therefore this book strives not to be theoretical but rather practical.

Only the first two chapters do not contain a description of specific clinical work with this population. The first chapter is the story of a man with AIDS who is in recovery from alcoholism and drug addiction. Having this individual tell his story in his own words is an excellent introduction to the complexities of doing this work. The second chapter by Dr. Iris Davis is an introduction to the varieties of medical problems of people who are both chemically dependent and infected with HIV. This way non-medical counselors and therapists can have a preliminary understanding of what their patients might physiologically be undergoing.

Each of the other chapters contain actual case material that illustrates what each author is discussing. In addition to the specific chapters focusing on work with clients who are members of ethnic minorities, many of the cases reported in most of the chapters reflect work with people of the inner city, women as well as men. This is tremendously important since so many chemically dependent individuals with HIV illness are minority individuals. But the cases contained in this volume are also about work with non-minority people, both gay and heterosexual. This is important because all too often there is the assumption and bias that only poor people of color are addicted to drugs. One case presented by Fontaine is about the difficulties of working with a white lesbian on an outpatient basis who is chronically relapsing into active drug use.

Two of the articles might be viewed as controversial by some in the drug treatment field. I am referring to Fontaine's article on outpatient therapy and Springer's article on prevention techniques. Both authors discuss their work with people who are *not* committed to abstinence from drug or alcohol use. This is a population that is desperately in need of the services described in this book and who are all too often prevented from accessing services since they can not or do not choose to refrain from using alcohol or drugs. Neither author is condoning continued drug use; they are both simply acknowledging that this population exists and are offering suggestions for drug treatment professionals and agencies attempting to work with both these clients' active chemical dependency and their HIV illness.

Many of the articles in this volume overlap with issues raised by others in this same volume. Several people briefly discuss how difficult they find doing this work, and the chapter by Chackes et al. on countertransference seeks to help workers address just this problem in a professional way.

One hope is that by reading this volume you will feel less isolated in the work you are doing with this population. If an article spoke to you particularly strongly as being relevant to your work, please share it with your colleagues. Also please feel free to contact any of the authors to discuss their work or to call upon them to come to your agencies to conduct staff trainings.

Someone once said that a society can be judged by how it treats it's most disadvantaged citizens. Contemporary American society has not for the most part demonstrated a significant level of caring for poor people, ethnic and sexual minorities, and people who are chemically dependent. I hope that this volume is one small step to improve the quality of care that chemically dependent people with

HIV illness receive from our health care and drug treatment professionals and institutions.

REFERENCES

Marmor, M., DesJarlais, D., Friedman S. et al. (1984). "The epidemic of acquired immunodeficiency syndrome (AIDS) and suggestions for its control in drug abusers." *Journal of Substance Abuse and Treatment*, 1, 237-247.

Siegel, L. (Ed). (1988). *AIDS and Substance Abuse*, New York: Harrington Park Press.

Being in Recovery and Having Aids

Peter S.

My name is Peter, I'm an alcoholic and a drug addict, and I have AIDS. This chapter tells how I became an alcoholic and drug addict, how I got sober, and what it's like to have AIDS in recovery. I believe the disease of AIDS and the diseases of alcoholism and drug addiction are inextricably tied to one another. This then, is my story, the same one I have shared with my sponsor and in A.A. meetings so many times. I hope that this helps your work with persons with AIDS who are in recovery from alcoholism and drug addiction.

I was born fifty-two years ago in the front seat of my father's car. My mother went into labor suddenly and my father drove to the nearest hospital. By the time he got there, I was almost born. He rushed in to tell the emergency room staff that his wife was having a baby outside in the car. When he rushed back to the car and opened the front door, I popped out and he caught me "like a football," as he told me years later. I weighed 10 lbs. 11 oz. but was placed in an incubator because of the evening chill in the air. I had a slight case of pneumonia and was kept in the hospital for several weeks. Six months later I developed pneumonia again. When I was ten years old, I had imphanema (pus around the lungs). When I was in the Army at age 21, I had pneumonia and 108 fever, and then years later in New York, I almost died from another bad bout of bacterial pneumonia. All of this no doubt weakened my natural defenses against disease and infection. But not nearly as much as alcohol and drugs were to do later in my life.

Neither of my parents were alcoholics, yet there was alcoholism in our family. My mother's brother who lived across the street from us was a raging alcoholic who killed himself when he split his head open on a radiator. He was found in a pool of beer, broken glass,

5

and blood by one of my aunts. I suspect that one of my mother's uncles also had a problem with alcohol and gambling. He didn't come around very often, and my mother wouldn't discuss it. But we knew he lived and worked at the YMCA on Skid Row.

There was very little alcohol kept in our house. What alcohol there was, was kept in the basement and was rarely brought out even for guests. There were rarely guests, as my mother didn't like having company over, and she hated when people drank liquor.

I had a difficult time growing up. My parents were middle-aged when they had my sister and me, so there was a tremendous gap between my parents and us. It was like being raised by grandparents, neither of whom had the strength or patience to deal with a rebellious child. From the time I was born, my mother had mental and emotional difficulties in dealing with my sister and me. She was a terrible housekeeper. There was always a lot of screaming and yelling and sometimes she threw things at us, like knives or whatever else was handy.

As far back as I can remember, I slept in the front bedroom with my father in a double bed, and my sister slept in a double bed with my mother in the rear bedroom. The middle bedroom was filled with singing canaries that my father raised as a hobby. The basement was also filled with canaries.

My mother accidentally killed them all one year when she put too much coal on the stoker, causing the house to fill up with smoke. My father wouldn't speak to her for six months, and we always thought she did it on purpose because she didn't want him to have birds in the house. He spent very little time with my sister and me. He left the task of raising us mainly to my mother, but she was not really capable of handling us. My parents fought, and yelled, and argued a lot, and came close to separating more than once, though they never did. In fact they lived on into very old age and mellowed considerably towards one another in their later years together.

My father was very strict with me, and I was always getting into trouble. When I was only four or five, I took a whole pack of Camel cigarettes from my father's things and went and smoked the whole pack with a friend in the alley. When I came home sick, they figured out that I had taken the cigarettes, but I don't think they believed I smoked them all. At age 12 I began to smoke on a regular basis and continued until I was 32 years old. When I quit, I was smoking four packs a day, plus five to ten joints of grass. I quit cigarettes, but not the grass.

When I was ten years old I discovered and promptly stole a fifth of gin from the cabinet in the basement. I drank the whole bottle with a friend my age, roaming the streets of our neighborhood until I finally walked into a moving car. I hit the car, rather then being hit by it. I said I was OK to the driver, and he let me go. I staggered home and my sister met me at the door and helped to the bathroom and held my head over the toilet when I threw up. My parents were out and never found out about this incident. I don't remember having another drink until I was in high school.

I knew from about age 10 that I was very different from the other kids my age since I was sexually attracted to other boys and men. I had heard that this was not normal, and thus I grew up with a big secret.

In school I was interested in subjects that my parents considered superficial or even worthless. I excelled in art, music, and writing, subjects my parents said didn't count. They wanted me to concentrate on arithmetic and science, despite the fact that I hated them. I did not believe my parents about a lot things since many of the things they tried to teach my sister and me were so absurd that, even as children, we knew they were not true. For example, they told us, "You don't have to brush your teeth since you're going to lose them when you grow up. Then you'll have to get false teeth." Both my parents had complete dentures.

As I grew older, the gap between my parents and me grew bigger. My sister excelled in school and skipped a year. From then on she was held up to me as a superior example of how I should be in every way. I was repeatedly told that I was no good and that I was "a bum" who would never amount to anything. This was because I was "so bull-headed" or stubborn, according to my parents. My report card reflected this, I got poor grades in everything except art and music. I was always scolded for not paying attention and for being a difficult student with unsatisfactory conduct. Frankly I didn't care. I began to do things my own way because "they" didn't know what they were talking about. I plunged into the music of Schoenberg, Stravinsky, Hindemith, and Barber. I took myself to the Art Institute and fell in love with Picasso and the post-Impressionists. By high school my parents as well as teachers knew I was different. They still didn't understand me. And I resented them greatly.

I remember my father being physically violent with me from an early age for almost anything he called a house rule, or if my report card was bad, which it was most of the time. I went to Catholic schools from grammar school through college. At that time, the nuns used corporal punishment. The priests in high school resorted to a combination of physical retribution and psychological intimidation. I had a terrible time just staying in school. I didn't want to listen to anyone in authority.

Yet in high school I met and was confronted by a teacher who turned my life around. He asked why I was having such a difficult time. He told me he thought I was very bright and doing well in school should be easy for me. I don't know why that made such a difference, or why I heard it, but I did.

I went from having terrible grades and being on probation to the top of my class. In my senior year, I was to give the valedictory address. Despite my academic turnaround, my parents continued to tell me I would never make it and that I should quit school and go to work in a factory to earn a living and pay my own way.

During this period, I was openly defiant of almost everything they said and told me to do. They said I'd never finish school. I showed them by graduating at the top of my class. When I said I wanted to go away to college, their response was, "You'll never get accepted, and how will you pay for it? We're not going to support you." I did get accepted and worked in a factory every summer to pay my way through college. When I was accepted on a graduate scholarship to a prominent Ivy League school, they were thunderstruck. They gave themselves all the credit for the good job they had done with me.

All during my adolescence, I was unhappy and in a lot of psychic pain. I knew that my parents didn't understand me, and I thought no one else understood me either. No one knew about my awakening sexual feelings for other boys and men. I was told I was no good and would never amount to anything. Why couldn't I be more like my sister who was so bright and clever, a near perfect daughter. I would "never have a dime" because I would spend it all. I also heard from my parents that I would have to do something to control the anger I constantly let out because it would get me into trouble.

I moved away from home to go to college. That began my serious drinking which spanned over thirty years. I had a great capacity for beer, and I really enjoyed getting drunk as it got me away from my pain and unhappiness. Being drunk was the only thing that made me feel powerful and not different. It was during these periods of drunkenness in college that I had my first blackouts. Drinking also helped me cover up the fact that I was attracted to many of my school mates and wanted to act on these sexual feelings. Since I didn't even feel comfortable having homosexual feelings, there was no way I could have approached another man at that point in my life. So instead I proceeded to get drunk a lot both to block out the uncomfortable feelings I was having as well as to numb myself to my growing frustration about not having any sexual outlets.

After a year of graduate school in the East, I decided I wanted to move to New York and be an actor. But first I had to get the Army out of the way. After six months in the National Guard, I moved to New York and began a life in the theater. Once I moved to New York I felt free to do things my way, and that meant getting drunk quite often if not every day.

Two things that characterized that period of my life were hangovers and blackouts. The hangovers would leave me totally debilitated for days following a binge. The blackouts were very serious. Often, I found myself waking up in a stranger's bed not knowing how I got there. Or I would wake up in my own apartment and literally not remember anything of what had happened the night before.

I had some affairs with women when I was in college. When I came to New York, I had an affair with the woman who lived next door and made her pregnant. She had an abortion in the days before abortion was legalized. It was a horrible experience for both of us, and she almost died from it. After she recuperated, I went to Minnesota to do summer stock. A week after I arrived, I came out sexually with another young leading man in the company. We bought a bottle of rum the first weekend before the season opened and drove out into the country and proceeded to get very drunk and have sex.

When I returned to New York, I really came out and began exploring all the places that gay men met one another at the time; certain streets where men who wanted to have sex with other men met, Central Park, gay bars, and public rest rooms.

In 1965 I discovered drugs by smoking marijuana. Soon afterwards I began to use pills. It didn't matter what they were as long as they got me high. This was when I also discovered acid, mescaline, and M.D.A. I thought drugs were terrific since I never suffered from hangovers after using them.

Beginning in the late 60's I also got involved in leather as a sexual fantasy and fetish. Drugs and leather seemed to fit together. The drugs made it easier for me to live out the various leather sex fantasies and seemed to endow this kind of sex with a certain power.

In 1968 I got a job in the business end of theater, and my intake of hallucinagenics and marijuana increased. I got involved with someone who was a dealer, which I thought was wonderful. It was like living in a candy store. Every summer for the next five years was an orgy of drugs and sex at Fire Island. I did not believe I had a problem with drugs or alcohol. Life was simply about living for the next sex scene or the next party.

On Fire Island in 1972 I did "angel dust" for the first time and had a bad trip. Two weeks later I went back to Fire Island and had another bad trip without taking any drugs. The people I was with left me alone and I went completely psychotic in their house. A neighbor talked me down off the roof as I was about to jump and called another friend who came and got me and took me back to his house. But instead of getting better, I began to hallucinate even more and became violent. Someone called the police, and I was taken off the island in a straight jacket. I fought and spit and bit the police. They took me to a state mental hospital on Long Island, where I was admitted overnight. The next day my boyfriend, the dealer, got me released to his psychiatrist. I swore I'd never do drugs again. Except maybe a little grass to smooth me out, and I promptly went back to drinking. Drinking didn't cause these kind of problems.

Shortly after this incident, I lost a very good job in the arts because of drugs. I thought everyone was against me, and I decided it was time to leave New York. I began a series of moves around the country to different cities in different jobs. Four years later I was back in New York with no job. Somewhere along the way, I had discovered one of the great loves of my life: Jack Daniels bourbon.

In 1977 I met my present lover in a New York bar along the waterfront. On our first night, we did more cocaine than I had ever done before. The second night we did even more, and I asked how he could afford to be so generous. "Easy," he told me. He supported his habit by dealing. I said to myself, "This boy really has a problem, and I'm going to help him. I'm going to get him to stop doing cocaine."

Next time we met I decided to confront him. I told him *he* had a problem and asked if he thought he could stop. He said yes, he certainly could. And he did, for a while. We began seeing each other exclusively and soon became lovers.

Ten years later we were both still doing cocaine, and I had developed a habit as big as or bigger than my lover's. But in addition to drugs, my drinking had increased considerably.

With the advent of AIDS, we decided to have a sexually exclusive relationship, which we have to this day. Early on in the epidemic a friend of ours was diagnosed, and we took part in caring for him. By 1983 I was deeply involved in GMHC, and for the next two and a half years, I cared for many people with AIDS and did many hours of volunteer work every week. This involvement in caring for other people seemed to control my alcohol and drug intake for awhile. As I began to burnout in 1986 I used speed to get through the long days and nights. I used Jack Daniels to take the edge off the speed. I also used it to numb myself to all of the loss and the sense of betrayal that I was feeling. The only way I was able to fall asleep each night was by drinking and taking Valium. I thought if I didn't have a night cap, I wouldn't be able to sleep. I was experiencing a lot of pain. Alcohol and drugs seemed to be the only things that helped.

In 1986 my lover got a job that was very time consuming. His employer supplied drugs to keep people working around the clock. I felt abandoned and betrayed, and I drank to numb myself to these feelings. By this time, my drinking had progressed further than I cared to admit. My drug intake was primarily, but not exclusively, limited to cocaine and amphetamines. I used Valium or Tuinal to bring me down, "smooth me out," or to knock me out.

In 1987 I was offered and accepted a job in AIDS education that was a tremendous professional opportunity. The problem was that I was strung out on drugs and beginning to have physical symptoms that I couldn't figure out. I had sweats almost all the time, and I was very paranoid about everything and almost everyone. Most of all I was afraid that my drug and alcohol problem would be discovered, and as a result, I would lose my new job.

Out of fear and desperation I had a consultation with a therapist I knew from my work at GMHC. During our first session, he suggested I go to Alcoholic's Anonymous. I did and hated it at first. But soon I realized these people had something very precious, something I wanted. At first I wanted to do it my way; for three months I had no sponsor to guide me and I kept using cocaine. I found out I was very sneaky with drugs. I was keeping one day count for alcohol and another one for drugs.

Finally, approaching my fiftieth birthday, I became "clean and dry," learning to be truly sober one day at a time. I was starting to get better physically, too. My life had finally begun to become manageable. Everyone I knew both in and out of AA told me I looked so much better. A week after my ninety days (which was also my fiftieth birthday), I was out in the sun too long and I developed a slight case of shingles on my neck. It was enough to send me running to the doctor, since I knew that it was a possible harbinger of HIV infection. I wanted to have all the necessary information about my health and took the HIV test that week. Two weeks later I found out that I was HIV +. I felt confident I could deal with it using the tools I was learning in AA. Having gotten sober, I knew that anything was possible.

Then my energy level dramatically decreased, and I would have trouble getting through the day without a nap. My doctor began monitoring my immune system, and it became apparent (to me) that I was very immune compromised. My T cells were just under 200, and I still had the sweats, especially at night. My doctor kept telling me not to worry. I asked him why I wasn't on a prophylaxis for PCP. He said we had to "get a better baseline." In late December I switched to another doctor, who put me on prophylaxis immediately.

In early January I got very sick with what turned out to be viral meningitis. In one 24 hour period, I was given 1 million units of penicillin and two other antibiotics which knocked out the meningitis but also seemed to have permanently damaged my intestinal tract. From the time that I was released from the hospital, I began to experience profound diarrhea, and I was hospitalized four times for gastro-intestinal problems. For the last six months, I have been undergoing treatment successfully to control the diarrhea. I am back to work full time and doing quite well.

So here I am, two and half years later, living with AIDS one day at a time and staying clean and dry, one day at a time. In a certain sense, I've never been better off in my life. First of all I'm sober and drug free after all those years, and things are so different now because of that alone. I'm the first one in the office every morning. I love my work and the people I work with. I no longer live in fear of losing my job, and I have become tremendously respected in my field. I respect my body and take as good care of it as I possibly can. I go to a yoga class for people with AIDS, and I've even begun to exercise at home. I attend a weekly support group for persons with AIDS. I still go to the therapist that got me into AA.

I know that the only reason I am able to deal with my diagnosis with serenity and hopefulness is because I'm clean and dry. I go to five or six AA meetings a week, including special meetings only for people who are HIV positive or who have AIDS. I also work my AA program by giving service to other people in the program. Currently I am chairing a Step meeting every week. I also have begun working in the soup kitchen of my church every Sunday.

The principles of AA have helped me more than anything else to deal with having AIDS. About a year and a half ago, I went to my first special interest HIV+/AIDS AA meeting. It was held in the living room of George N., the man who started the first meeting of this kind in NYC. Walking in to that meeting, I was terribly anxious and scared. By the end of the meeting, I was drained and yet I felt wonderfully exhilarated as well. There were a dozen men, mostly gay, and one black woman at that meeting. I identified completely with the feelings each of these people shared. I heard many differing views and opinions about AIDS treatments and what people were doing to deal with their situations. Like at most AA meetings, there were tears and laughter.

It was important for me to hear people talk about hope and gratitude. But most important, these people had one more thing in common. They were all living sober with HIV and AIDS. At the end of the meeting, I hugged every person there. That meeting made a deep and lasting impression on me.

That meeting grew from ten to over forty people or more within a matter of months. Shortly after that some friends and I started another HIV+/AA meeting downtown in the Village. We started out in one person's apartment, then moved to another, and finally found a space to have meetings that was not in someone's apartment.

These meetings are very special to me because I can go and talk about my HIV disease and hear things that other people with HIV/AIDS are dealing with. I can talk AIDS openly and not be self-conscious.

Talking about AID's at a regular AA meeting can be awkward. People come up to you after the meeting and say things like, "Do you have a good doctor? Is he connected to a good hospital? You're sure you're alright?" Once someone came up asked, "How does it feel to know you're dying?" Usually they mean well, but it can be very uncomfortable.

Once when I was sick in the hospital, I asked my sponsor to set up a meeting for me in my room. It was wonderful, like a warm healing ray of sunshine for my body and soul. When I came home from the hospital, I was confined to my apartment, so I had some AA meetings in my apartment. These were a wonderful source of comfort. There is nothing quite like a meeting for someone who is in the Fellowship. The last time I came home from the hospital, the first thing I did was call someone to arrange a meeting in my apartment. The next morning a half dozen people showed up and we had a regular AA meeting. It was more healing to me than anything I know of, including massages, meditation or medicine.

Having AIDS and learning to live with it, a day at a time, has not been easy. What has helped me more than anything else is the AA program. Using the tools of AA I live soberly with AIDS, just one day at a time. I give my life and my will over to the care of a Higher

Power that I call God. Knowing that I am doing the best I can, has given me the courage to deal with the things I have to face. I don't know why I'm still here. By all rights I should be dead and buried. I have come face to face with death many times, and yet I'm still alive. It's all part of a bigger picture, God's plan. I have faith that whatever happens, I won't have to go through it alone. No matter what happens, me and my Higher Power are going to handle it together. And as long as I don't pick up a drink or a drug, I know everything else will be alright, one day at a time.

What Drug Treatment Professionals Need to Know About Medical Aspects of HIV Illness

Iris Davis, MD

The dual diagnosis of Human Immunodeficiency Viral Disease (HIV) and substance abuse disorders is a critical interface in American medicine today. The combined prevalence of these diseases is not definitively known, but must be estimated since they are primarily measured by those with significant end stage disease in both of these chronic conditions. The increasing caseload of individuals with chemical dependency who are now presenting to the health care system for treatment of their substance abuse disorder, HIV disease, or other medical disorders have increased in such numbers in recent years that our health system, both ambulatory and hospital-based, is overwhelmed by the numbers and needs. The needs of these patients are not easily met, frequently due to the type of services available and training of staff in institutions where individuals receive ambulatory care. As the knowledge base expands concerning HIV disease, categories of substance abuse that place individuals at risk for HIV disease continue to grow.

Since in its early phases, HIV is a primarily asymptomatic illness, many patients will present on an ambulatory basis. An ambulatory patient can be defined as such when an individual presents for "personal health services who is neither bedridden nor currently admitted to any health care institution" (Barker, 1991). Ambulatory patients are usually responsible for the majority of their care (e.g., taking their own medication, monitoring their symptoms, and following their response to treatment). Primary or ambulatory care should be coordinated with all factors necessary for health maintenance including comprehensive medical care and social services necessary to support good health.

Although the majority of HIV infected individuals will present as above, those who have co-morbidity due to chemical dependency may arrive at acute care institutions because of complications from their drug or alcohol use, lack of primary care services in many economically disadvantaged areas, or because of being at a symptomatic stage of HIV disease. Unless these individuals are extremely endstage or die of their acute illness, eventually they will also need integration into a system of ambulatory or primary care where they can be maintained in the community. The implications of the above presentations will be discussed later.

DEFINITION AND VIROLOGY

HIV disease is a chronic, eventually fatal immune cell destructive disease. After the onset of viral infection, the course of the disease can remain asymptomatic for extremely long periods (as long as 10 years in some individuals), and each infected person acts as a potential reservoir for continuing infection to others. The extended stage of asymptomatic infection has a tremendous impact on the changing epidemiology of the disease.

EPIDEMIOLOGY

Statistics of HIV seroprevalence in the American population are not definitively known. Presently, estimations vary from one to one and a half million infected people in the United States (Quinn, 1991). AIDS has caused the death of over 100,000 Americans (CDC, 1991), which is sobering considering that these statistics reflect HIV infection from 5 to 10 years ago. By early 1991, 161,288 AIDS cases were reported. Ninety-eight per cent were adults; 1.7% were children under the age of 13 (CDC, 1991). By viewing the groups of "risk behavior," we can further delineate the multiple subepidemics that are changing the face of AIDS.

Presently the bulk of AIDS cases are male (90.8%); women comprise a much smaller group (9.2%) (CDC, 1991). Most individuals were between 20 to 50 years of age and mortality was significant at the initial point of reporting (55%) (Quinn, 1991). Five years after diagnosis, AIDS mortality was greater than 90%. The bulk of cases were due to sexual transmission (male to male type), but in certain areas of the country, intravenous drug use has superseded this means as the leading type of risk behavior for AIDS. For individuals who had a history of substance abuse, breakdown of mortality rates showed an even higher rate of mortality compared to males with a history of same sex contact as their only risk behavior. In addition, there were racial differences in mortality within each sub-group, with blacks and hispanics dying faster than white males (Quinn, 1991).

Reflecting trends of intravenous drug use in this country, AIDS cases are disproportionately higher in black and hispanic populations in the United States. Twenty-five per cent of all male cases are black and 15% hispanic. For women, the proportions are even more skewed since 52% of all female cases are black and 21% hispanic. The representative proportions of the total American population is 11.6% for blacks and 6.5% for hispanics. Blacks account for 53% of all pediatric cases and hispanics account for 25% of pediatric cases. AIDS is now one of the top five causes of death for both males and females between the ages of 20-44 in the United States (CDC, 1991).

The rate of AIDS in individuals who have a history of intravenous drug use or are sexual partners of individuals with a history of intravenous drug use but no male to male sexual contact increased from 14% of all AIDS cases nationally in 1987 to 20% of all cases by 1988. The proportion of women who have never used intravenous drugs, but had sexual partners at risk increased from 15% of all females in 1984 to 20% in 1991. This heterosexual transmission group forms the fastest growing group among AIDS cases. If women who have a history of intravenous drug use and a partner who is an intravenous user are included, the percentage of possible sexual transmission increases as a major cause of HIV disease among women.

PATHOGENESIS AND NATURAL HISTORY

HIV-1 is the name of the virus that has been identified as causing illnesses related to AIDS. This virus depletes the body by affecting multiple important components of an individual's immune system.

This does not explain all the clinical phenomena we know as HIV disease because other diseases may act as cofactors and HIV affects other tissues in the body directly. The immune system component most frequently followed in clinical practice and considered to be most predictive of immune system disease is human T lymphocytes of the helper/inducer group. Other names for these cells are T4 cells or CD4 cells. These cells are critical for cell-mediated immunity, and their eventual destruction in HIV disease leads to the onset of opportunistic (usually non-pathogenic or not seen in normal immune function) infections that are the primary cause of death in HIV infection. Measurement of T4 cells is an important clinical indicator of immune suppression, and levels are used to initiate primary and prophylactic therapies. The normal range for T4 cells is above 500. When blood tests indicate that T4 cells have fallen below 500, this indicates that the immune system is compromised, and it is often suggested that an individual begin anti-retroviral therapy in the form of AZT.

CD4 Cell Count	Medical Followup
>600	Repeat CD4 each 6 months
500-600	Repeat CD4 every three months
200-500	Initiate retroviral therapy
< 200	Initiate pneumocystis carinii pneumonia prophylaxis

HIV Testing

HIV testing is based on the immune response of the body to the virus. Unlike other diseases, the antibody response to HIV is not curative but rather defines a chronic carrier state. The antibody response can usually be detected between four to twenty-four weeks after a person has been exposed to the virus, although there is a very small subpopulation who may remain seronegative for longer periods of time.

HIV diagnosis is based on two tests—the ELISA and the Western Blot. Tests are reported as positive or negative for ELISA; the Western Blot is reported as positive, negative, or indeterminate. ELISA tests are reported as having sensitivity (true positive results out of the total population) of 99% and specificity (number of true negatives of all negative results in a population) of 99.5%. False positives occur when patients have other immunologic abnormalities, such as connective tissue disorders (lupus, rheumatoid arthritis). False negatives can be seen in populations that have not yet seroconverted.

Indeterminate Western Blots may mean that a person is seroconverting, or it may not indicate HIV infection. After six months, if this pattern remains stable, further evaluation such as viral culture or other specialized tests should be utilized and can usually be obtained through a local department of health or academic medical center.

Because of the possibility of a severe response to a positive HIV test, varying from depression and suicide to an increase in drug using behavior,and also because of a frequent lack of knowledge about asymptomatic HIV illness or treatment, counseling is important. Privacy should be insured for both pretest and post-test counseling and adequate time allotted, even if more than one provider or frequent revisits are required to complete this goal. Small studies have shown that the behavior and perceived attitude of the providers are important in the patient's decision to return for test results and follow-up and in how the test result is perceived (Rugg, 1990).

Negative attitudes and assumptions of medical providers have been documented concerning substance abusers and HIV positive individuals (Sadovsky, 1989). Yet multiple studies document that individuals with a history of drug abuse will seek medical treatment and that compliance can be equal to or improved over other populations for drug treatment, HIV treatment and appointments. In fact, some substance abusers may never stop use of drugs but will come in for other medical treatment so compliance with medical treatment is not necessarily compromised by drug using behavior (Davis, 1989).

CLINICAL SYNDROMES

The Centers for Disease Control (CDC) published a classification system in the late 1980's for HIV disease which set a worldwide standard for "AIDS." See Figure 1. It is important to remember that clinical disease does not always correlate with CDC definition and that the classification system will continue to evolve over years as severe HIV disease that does not presently fit the criteria is better defined. Presently, individuals with a history of substance abuse, minorities, and women have a higher incidence of dying with HIV disease that does not fit the CDC criteria.

FIGURE 1

```
       STAGES   OF   HIV   INFECTION
       STAGE                *TIME                     CLINICAL
SYMPTOMS
Acute                    4 - 24 weeks        viral like syndrome
Seroconversion                               meningitis, rash
Asymptomatic             2 - 10 years        generalized
                                             lymphadenopathy
Symptomatic              3-24 months         oral thrush, anemia,
                                             thrombocytopenia,
                                             herpes zoster,
                                             increased bacterial
                                             infections, cervical
                                             dysplasia
Advanced HIV Disease     12 - 24 months      CDC defined AIDS,
                                             multiple severe
                               infections, neoplasms
              *Time is based on mean statistics.
```

Management and Evaluation

Initially, patients require a full evaluation to serve as a baseline for future evaluation and provide key information to determine early intervention. This should include extensive clinical and laboratory data.

A full review of systems should include at least the following symptoms:

- *constitutional*: history of weight loss, fever, night sweats or swollen lymph nodes
- *skin*: rashes or lesions; a history of herpes zoster (shingles)
- *Head, ear, nose and throat*: a change in vision, unusual headaches, lesions or a white coating of the tongue or mouth; ulcers of the mouth
- *respiratory (lungs)*: shortness of breath
- *gastrointestinal (stomach)*: difficulty swallowing, diarrhea, a history of hepatitis, rectal cramping
- *neuropsychiatric*: depression, memory loss, painful limbs or weakness
- *genitourinary*:discharge (penile or vaginal); recurrent genital infections, recurrent candidiasis in women; history of abnormal PAP smear, a history of any sexually transmitted disease;

lifelong partner history (male or female) and partner preference; number of pregnancies

Acute Infection

This portion of the infection is often misinterpreted as a flu-like syndrome. One study found that up to 75% of seroconverters could identify the syndrome (Tindall, 1991). The syndrome usually lasts for 24 hours to three months, with an incubation period of two to four weeks.

Asymptomatic Follow-Up Care

Individuals who are without symptoms will receive their medical care based on their CD4 cell counts. Antiretroviral therapy such as zidovudine (AZT) is the primary method of treatment for HIV disease in this country. Important issues concerning retroviral medication or any treatment in HIV disease are a lack of data for substance using populations or populations on methadone. A small recently released study from the Veteran's Administration questioned the efficacy of AZT in minority populations; however, a second review of the data continued to show decreased morbidity for those individuals on AZT (ACTG release).

Many individuals with a history of chemical dependence have liver disease which is important since the liver is the primary organ responsible for clearance of the family of drugs. Therefore, these individuals may be extremely limited in their choices of treatment for HIV disease. Other types of agents that may be used for HIV disease should be considered and may be experimental. Experimental protocols are available for HIV disease through the national trials system and many medical complexes where HIV research is done. If clients have limited access or need further information, they can call 1-800-TRIALS or contact local or national HIV service organizations. Due to frequent chronic medical disorders seen in chemically dependent populations or refusal to allow people who continue to actively use illicit drugs into research trials, patients with a history of chemical dependency are severely underrepresented in AIDS clinical research trials (Long, 1990).

Tuberculosis Prevention

Since the HIV pandemic has been noted, the previously dropping rates for tuberculosis in this country are now rising primarily in areas where HIV is endemic. These areas include New York, New Jersey, Florida, and California. Persons more likely to have both HIV disease and tuberculous disease are minority, Haitian, homeless, or intravenous drug users. The diagnosis of tuberculosis is an important component of the medical care of individuals who have a history of substance abuse. In populations that have a high rate of tuberculous exposure such as intravenous drug users, those with HIV disease have a greater incidence of active tuberculosis (Selwyn, 1989).

All patients with HIV disease or suspected risk behavior for HIV disease should be tested for tuberculosis to receive early preventive therapy.

Vaccinations

The majority of individuals with HIV disease will benefit from vaccinations. The following schedule of vaccinations is recommended:

- Pneumococcal vaccine (for pneumonia)
- Hepatitis B vaccine for those not previously exposed
- Influenza vaccine yearly
- Measles booster if applicable

Pneumocystis carinii prophylaxis

Sixty per cent of AIDS patients are diagnosed as having AIDS due to pneumonia from pneumocystis infection. In addition, 20% of all AIDS patients who were diagnosed as having AIDS based on other diseases will develop pneumonia due to pneumocystis. Some patients will have more than one episode. Pneumocystis is still the most common cause of death in AIDS patients. All patients who have a CD4 cell count of 200 or less or an abnormal ratio of CD4 cells to the total lymphocyte count of less than 20% should be started on therapy to decrease the disease due to this organism. There are multiple therapies for preventing this disease, and they include oral drugs such as Bactrim (trimethoprim-sulfamethox-azole) or dapsone and pentamidine which is inhaled through a nebulizer once monthly.

COMPLICATIONS AND SPECIFIC INFECTIONS

Dermatologic or Skin Disorders

Skin disease is a common complication of HIV disease, occurring in up to 90% of cases (Berger, 1991). Common dermatologic conditions that are seen and are often more severe in HIV infected individuals are seborrheic dermatitis, psoriasis, ichthyosis (dry skin), and infections. The infections may be bacterial, mycobacterial (tuberculous), fungal, or viral. HIV seropositive individuals can also demonstrate an increased sensitivity to the sun and have an increased incidence of drug hypersensitivity reactions which involve the skin.

Many of the dermatologic conditions can be noted when an individual is asymptomatic, e.g., shingles or herpes zoster, both of which can be very painful. Shingles are a significant sign of immunosuppression and should alert the health practitioner to consider HIV testing and counseling.

Mouth Complications

Lesions of the mouth are frequently the harbinger of the immunosuppression caused by HIV disease. The most common problem is thrush or candidiasis, a common fungal infection that appears as a white coating of the tongue, lining of the mouth, or throat. Five to ten percent of patients have thrush within the first six months of being seropositive and between 33% to 50% of HIV positive individuals will have thrush eventually (Horn, 1991). Candida can also cause a breakdown of the corners of the mouth known as angular cheilosis or redness of the tongue. Thrush is important to note since the presence of thrush indicates a likelier progression to AIDS.

Another common disorder is oral hairy leukoplakia. This lesion is secondary to viral infection, most likely, and presents as a shaggy appearing white coating on the lateral aspects of the tongue. It may appear like thrush, but diagnostic tests are negative for fungus. This lesion is also an indication of immunosuppression and should be an indication to obtain HIV testing and counseling in non-diagnosed cases.

Although an individual may have good oral hygiene, inflammation of the gums or gingivitis can be a significant problem. Cancers such as Kaposi's sarcoma or other opportunistic infections may also initially appear in the mouth of persons who have been infected with HIV.

Disorders of the Nervous System

Ten per cent of patients with AIDS present initially with neurologic disease. By the point of death, over 75% of patients will have some type of neurologic involvement. By late stages of infection, up to 65% of patients have AIDS dementia complex which has specific diagnostic findings. These may present as symptoms such as depression, memory loss, and mood swings. In order for an individual to be diagnosed with AIDS dementia, other diseases of the central nervous system (the brain) must be excluded first. When AIDS dementia is suspected in early stages, neuropsychological testing may be required.

Some of the common opportunistic infections that affect the central nervous system include cryptococcal meningitis, toxoplasma, lymphoma, tuberculosis, and cryptococcus. One disease that may cause isolated symptoms or present as a focal mass is progressive multifocal leukoencephalopathy. This is a disorder that strips the brain of important proteins (myelin). This condition progresses over weeks or months, usually until the patient is severely compromised and eventually dies.

Because of the frequent subtle presentations of these diseases, small symptoms should not be lightly considered. Most often patients will present with fever and headache, but some patients may have no warning signs. Some patients may have experience seizures as the first symptom of brain-related HIV illnesses.

HIV can also infect the cells of the peripheral nervous system. When the cells of the peripheral nervous system are affected a patient may suffer from neuropathies, which are pains in the limbs or difficulty in walking. Opportunistic infections also can cause the same symptoms and drugs may easily exacerbate or "unmask" neuropathy.

Psychiatric Manifestations

This may be one of the most challenging areas in working with some HIV infected patients. Certainly, a psychiatric disorder can predate the diagnosis of HIV illness. Learning of seropositive diagnosis alone can cause severe stress and depression, as can having to cope with the manifestations of the disease. It is important to rule out neurologic causes for all new psychiatric disorders in HIV infected patients, such as psychosis, paranoia, or even apathy, mental slowing, and depression. Treatment of these disorders should also be aggressive and use of antidepressants and other drugs should be appropriately initiated.

Complications of the Gastrointestinal System

The wasting syndrome is one of the most well-known symptoms of HIV disease and is now an AIDS defining illness. The criteria are based on significant involuntary weight loss (greater than 10% form baseline) in conjunction with either chronic diarrhea for at least 30 days or chronic weakness and fever. These symptoms must be in the absence of any other explanation, such as opportunistic infection, and can be complicated by an individual's actively abusing substances.

All parts of the gastrointestinal tract can be affected in HIV disease. One of the most common findings is that of esophagitis or disorders of the esophagus, the tube-like structure between the mouth and the stomach. Typical symptoms of esophagitis are difficulty in swallowing or painful swallowing and is most commonly due to Candida infection. When a person is diagnosed with Candida esophagitis, not oral thrush, he fits the criteria for an AIDS defining illness. Other infectious agents that can infect the esophagus and cause similar symptoms are herpes virus and cytomegalovirus.

Liver disease is common in people with HIV infection as there is almost universal exposure to Hepatitis B disease in HIV infected individuals. Certain patterns of liver abnormalities must be evaluated to determine if opportunistic infections such as tuberculosis, usually the atypical type, fungal, or other viral infections are the cause of the abnormalities. Kaposi's sarcoma can often cause abnormalities of the liver or stomach.

Diarrheal disease is a significant problem in HIV disease affecting up to 50% of patients during the course of their disease (Horn, 1991). Two-thirds of the diarrhea is usually identifiable as due to some kind of illness-causing organism like intestinal parasites; the other third is usually attributed to HIV infection. Some patients require significant antidiarrheal medications, a few of which contain belladonna or morphine. For patients in drug treatment programs, this may sometimes cause a conflict with the goals of the program.

Respiratory Disease

The lung is the most common organ involved in opportunistic infections in HIV disease. Symptoms of PCP are usually less acute than other pneumonias, with slowly increasing shortness of breath, fever, night sweats, and cough usually without sputum production. All these symptoms may not be evident at the time when the pneumonia begins. Physical exam and even chest X-ray may not be helpful during the earlier stages of the pneumonia, so patients are often diagnosed by means of special radiologic studies (gallium scans), (Gram Weigert), an arterial blood gas (to measure oxygen capacity) and may even require a bronchoscopy, a procedure to obtain tissue and washings directly from the lungs. Treatment for the acute pneumonia is usually three weeks in length and is accomplished with the use of multiple drugs. Often, therapy is complicated by the high incidence of drug toxicity in patients. Without preventive therapy, 50 to 60% of patients will have a second episode a year after the first episode.

Other Complicating Illnesses

The predominant infection of the eyes is cytomegalovirus (CMV), seen in 20% of AIDS patients, which if not treated aggressively can lead to blindness. Treatment is lifelong and will usually require the placement of an catheter directly into a vein for daily intravenous infusion of medication. For patients who either are actively still using drugs intravenously or have a history of I. V. drug use, the surgical installation of a direct line to their veins can pose problems related to relapse.

CMV can also affect heart tissue leading to heart failure and arrhythmias (abnormal rhythms of the heart which can be fatal). HIV can directly affect the kidneys as well, leading to multiple abnormalities that can advance to renal failure.

Multiple blood abnormalities are seen in HIV disease whether from HIV itself, opportunistic infections affecting the bone marrow where blood cells arise, or from anemia caused by prescribed drugs — especially zidovudine (AZT).

SUMMARY

HIV disease can be manifested in a variety of symptoms. When an individual has had a history of intravenous drug use, he or she can present with a variety of illnesses that can complicate the diagnosis of HIV illness. It is critical for drug treatment professionals to have at least a rudimentary understanding of the medical conditions that their chemically dependent clients with HIV illness may be experiencing.

REFERENCES

Barker, L., Burton J. & Zieve P. (Eds). (1991). *Principles of Ambulatory Medicine*. Baltimore, MD: Williams and Wilkins.

Berger, T. (1991). "Dermatologic care in the AIDS patient." In M. Sande & P. Volberding (Eds.) *Medical Management of AIDS*, Philadelphia, PA: WB Saunders and Co, 114-130.

Centers for Disease Control. (1991). *AIDS*, 5(4), 473.

Davis, I. et al. (1989). "Evaluation of compliance rate in a clinic serving minority and low income communities." Fifth International Conference on AIDS.

Erickson J. (1990). "Examining risk for AIDS among minority intravenous drug users." Sixth International Conference on AIDS.

Horn, J., Yamaguchi, E., & Chiasson, R. (1991). "Ambulatory care for the HIV infected patient." In L. Barker, J. Burton J. & P. Zieve (Eds.), *Principles of Ambulatory Medicine*, Baltimore, MD: Wiliams and Wilkins, 375-397.

Long I., Davis I et al. (1990). "Demographic analysis of AIDS clinical treatment unit trial enrollment vs. incidence of AIDS in New York City." Sixth International Conference on AIDS.

MacCallum, L. (1990). "Assessment of Zidovudine use and concurrent opiate use." Sixth International Conference on AIDS.

National Institute of Allergies and Infectious Diseases AIDS Agenda Newsletter. 1991, 3-8.

Primm B., Brown L. et al. (1988) "The range of sexual behaviors of intravenous drug abusers." Fourth International Conference on AIDS.

Quinn T. (1991). "Global epidemiology of HIV infections." In M. Sande & P. Volberding (Eds). *Medical Management of AIDS*. Philadelphia, PA: WB Saunders and Co, 3-22.

Rugg, D. et al. (1989). "Why some do not return for their HIV test results." Fifth International Conference on AIDS.

Sadovsky R. (1989). "HIV-infected patients: a primary care challenge." *American Family Practice*, 121-128.

Tindall, B. et al. (1991). "Primary HIV infection." In M. Sande & P. Volberding, (Eds.). *Medical Management of AIDS*, Philadelphia, Pa: W. B. Saunders and Co.

Counseling Chemically Dependent HIV Positive Adolescents

William Reulbach, MSW

As the AIDS epidemic moves into the 1990s, public health officials are increasingly concerned that "the risk-related behaviors of adolescents puts some teenagers directly in the path of the epidemic." (Hein, 1989) Many of these at-risk youth are engaging in unprotected sexual intercourse (not using condoms) and substance abuse. In the next few years, larger numbers of at-risk adolescents will be referred for HIV antibody testing due to the increased benefits that have been associated with early treatment of asymptomatic HIV. Demands for comprehensive services for those who test positive will increase. These services must be designed to meet the unique needs of HIV positive adolescents. Now is the time for adolescent specialists from various disciplines to begin to prepare programs and strategies that will serve this special population. This paper will focus on an intervention strategy I developed for working with HIV positive substance abusing adolescents.

The strategy or treatment approach was developed within the context of an adolescent AIDS program at a large urban medical center. I was the social work member of a clinical treatment team consisting of a physician, nurse, social worker, outreach worker, and health educator. The clinical team provided comprehensive medical and psychosocial services to a caseload of thirty HIV positive and a larger number of at-risk adolescents between the ages of fourteen and twenty-one. This caseload can be understood as a "snapshot" of the epidemic within an urban adolescent population during 1989-90.

Recent statistics have demonstrated that HIV infection is already present in the United States adolescent population. The total number of reported cases of AIDS in persons thirteen to twenty-one years of age was 1,266 in October of 1989, or approximately one percent of the total cases of AIDS in the United States. Adults between the ages of twenty and twenty-nine, however, account for 21 percent of all the AIDS cases in the United States (Hein, 1990). Given the long incubation period of the virus from point of infection to the manifestation of first symptoms (estimated to be between eight to ten years on average), many of these adults were infected as adolescents (Hein, 1989).

The realization that the epidemic is indeed moving through the adolescent population has focused some attention on providing AIDS prevention and education programs that are targeted to young people. While it can be debated whether these programs have been effective, not enough attention has been paid to those adolescents who are already infected. I suspect that as the numbers of adolescents diagnosed with AIDS continues to grow and as the epidemic begins to move out of poor, minority, urban neighborhoods, increased attention and funding will be given to developing comprehensive adolescent focused programs and services. In the meantime adolescent based agencies and workers will need to adjust their programs and interventions to outreach and serve the HIV positive and at-risk adolescents who are already here. A knowledge of who these adolescents are is essential for the successful intervention and treatment.

Adolescence is normally a time of exploration, experimentation, and risk taking. Two such behaviors have increasingly become associated with the adolescent rite of passage: unprotected sexual intercourse and experimentation with drugs and alcohol. These same behaviors also put adolescents at-risk for acquiring HIV. The virus is transmitted through bodily fluids in oral, anal, and vaginal intercourse and through the sharing of virus contaminated needles in intravenous drug use (IVDU). However, other types of substance abuse can also put adolescents at increasing risk for possible infection. It is well known that alcohol and drugs can impair judgment and increase the likelihood that an adolescent might engage in risk behavior that they would have avoided if he or she were sober. In this way, substance abuse of all kinds can be understood as an additional risk factor if it prevents the adolescent from following safer-sex guidelines (using a condom). Adolescents who are at highest risk for HIV infection fall into four groupings: IVDUs, gay and bisexual males, those engaging in survival sex or sex-for-pay (prostitution), and those whose sex partners are or have engaged in these risk behaviors (Stiffman and Earls, 1990).

The majority of adolescents have been and will continue to be infected through unprotected sexual intercourse. Intravenous drug use in adolescence, unlike adulthood, accounts for only a small percentage of adolescent AIDS cases. Only 10 percent of all reported AIDS cases in adolescence were due to IVDU transmission. This rate, however, increases to 16 percent in males and 30 percent for female adolescents in New York City (Vermund, Hein et al., 1988). The rate of HIV infection among IVDUs is high. Estimates range all the way to 70 percent in some studies. In a New York City study it was estimated that 50 percent of IVDUs were infected.

Male adolescents who are engaging in unprotected male to male sex are also at high risk for infection because of the high rate of infection in the gay community (Drucker, 1986). The gay community has been remarkably effective in promoting safer sex guidelines among gays. Yet, some adolescents who are experimenting with male-to-male sex and do not consider themselves to be gay and gay adolescents who are isolated from the adult gay community often have not gotten this safer-sex message.

Adolescents who engage in survival sex are the third group who are at high risk for infection. There are approximately 1,000,000 homeless and runaway adolescents on the streets of America's urban centers at any one time. Many of them engage in sex-for-pay to buy food, drugs, shelter, and clothing, (Futterman, 1990). Crack use has also been associated with adolescent sex-for-pay as a means to exchange sex for or obtain money for crack (Fullilove and Fullilove, 1989). Crack is increasingly associated with HIV infection in adolescents (Futterman, Reuben et al., 1990). Because so many of the adolescents who engage in sex-for-pay are at the same time engaging in unprotected sexual intercourse and substance abuse, their risk is magnified by their number of encounters with high risk partners.

The majority of adolescents have been and will continue to be infected through unprotected sexual intercourse. The impact of this statement is realized in the escalating STD rates among adolescents.

Adolescents between the ages of thirteen and nineteen have the highest STD rates among any age group in the United States (Bell and Hein, 1984). Some studies have shown that one in seven adolescents between the ages of fifteen and nineteen get an STD every year. Some STDs may actually facilitate the transmission of virus through genitourinary ulcerative lesions (Futterman, 1990).

All four of these subgroupings were reflected in the client caseload in the adolescent AIDS program where I worked. For example, the demographics for twenty HIV positive adolescent clients followed in an ongoing study in the program are as follows: 13 male and 7 female; 8 Hispanic, 6 Afro-American, 4 White, and 3 Other. Seven of the males described themselves as gay, 3 as bisexual and 3 as heterosexual and all 7 females were heterosexual. Sixty percent of the sample were crack abusers before they tested positive. After testing positive 50 percent of this number stopped using crack (Futterman, Hein et al., 1990).

The other 50 percent who were still using crack and other drugs (some of this number also continued high risk sex-for-pay) were difficult to treat in the program. They were less likely to keep clinic appointments, follow through on health-promoting behaviors, e.g., taking medication or improving diet and practicing safer-sex guidelines than those adolescents who were not using drugs. They were also less likely to be able to negotiate the expected psychosocial counseling tasks of newly diagnosed HIV positive adolescents: to deal with the ambiguity of HIV positive diagnosis; integrate knowledge of HIV as a progressive, but gradual decline of the immune system; develop disclosure strategies for family and friends; make decisions regarding continuing sexual relationships and safer-sex practices, and in general, cope with the roller coaster emotions associated with HIV.

The case study which follows will illustrate some of the counseling dilemmas and frustrations that arise in working with HIV positive chemically dependent adolescents. There will be few surprises for those who are already familiar with working with a chemically dependent adolescent population. The treatment strategy I developed in working with this case is rather straight forward. Much of what I did is similar to other adolescent intervention strategies designed to motivate the adolescent to enter drug and alcohol treatment (Morehouse, 1989).

When I first met Carlos, he presented himself as a tough street kid. As I got to know him, I found him to be a frightened sixteen year old boy. He had just been released from a state youth detention center where he was placed after he was arrested for car theft when he was fifteen. During his last six months at the detention center, he had complained of swollen lymph glands under his arms. Eventually a biopsy was performed and it was determined that Carlos was HIV positive. Shortly thereafter, he was released back home. Carlos' probation officer referred him to the adolescent AIDS program.

At our first meeting, Carlos told me the story of his life in a matter of fact way that belied all of its tragic details. He has lived most of his life with his maternal grandmother because his mother abandoned him when he was five years old. Carlos' mother is a heroin addict, and although he sometimes sees her on the street, he doesn't speak to her. His grandmother is an alcoholic with a chronic heart problem. She has difficulty getting around and depends upon Carlos to help her with household tasks when he is home. Carlos never knew his father. His grandmother told him his father is in jail serving a life sentence for murder.

Carlos' earliest memory is being shot in the left eye with a pellet gun by a drunken uncle when he was four year old. He had to have several operations to repair the damage, and he endured years of disfigurement before he received a replacement glass eye. He was continually teased by other children at school. As he got older, he got into fights and finally dropped out of school in the eighth grade.

Eventually, Carlos drifted onto the streets. He started to hang out with a group of boys with whom he felt accepted and secure. They also turned him onto drugs. In the beginning, Carlos was happy hanging out and "partying" with his new-found friends. He drank a lot and smoked pot, but he promised himself that he would stay away from crack and heroin. He saw what the crack was doing to his friends, and he knew what the heroin did to his mother. Carlos doesn't remember why he smoked crack for the first time around his fifteenth birthday. He does know why he continues to smoke it: "It makes me feel better than I ever felt before."

As Carlos' drug abuse continued to increase, he experimented with a variety of drugs. His drug of choice remained crack. When he began to run out of ways to pay for the crack, a friend taught him how to hustle (prostitute) in a local park. Carlos found that hustling was the easiest way for him to get all the money he needed to support his crack habit. Carlos' good looks and outgoing personality made him very popular in the park. He also started to become addicted to the excitement and notoriety he got from hustling in the park. Before he was arrested, he was "scoring" ten to fifteen times a day with mainly anonymous older men who frequented the park. He was engaging in both unprotected oral and anal intercourse. This was undoubtedly how he became HIV infected.

Carlos had been sexually active with only two neighborhood girls before he started to hustle. As he became more drug involved, he only engaged in male-to-male sex. Carlos admits enjoying sex with men, but does not feel he is gay. His dream is to "marry a nice girl and have a family." A strong ethnic and social bias against homosexuality might be the cause of Carlos' confusion regarding his sexual identity.

During this first visit, Carlos claimed he had not smoked crack since he got out of the center. He admitted to drinking with some of his old friends, but felt that he was "strong" enough to stay away from the crack: "I know what it does to me and I don't want to go back to jail." He refused all my suggestions for drug treatment, insisting he could stay away from drugs on his own. Within a matter of weeks, Carlos was back in the park smoking crack and hustling sex.

Incredibly, Carlos kept all his clinic appointments during this time period. After his physical exams and tests were completed, Carlos' HIV positive diagnosis was confirmed, and he was found to be asymptomatic with an intact immune system. This meant that Carlos was, most likely, at the first stages of the infection and probably many years away from the earliest physical manifestations of the disease. From the beginning, Carlos had equated being HIV positive as having AIDS and a death sentence. Part of his medical management included extensive health education regarding the nature of HIV disease, stages in disease progression, advice on how to stay healthy and avoid infections to keep his immune system strong, and safer-sex practices. While Carlos seemed to take this all in, he continued to use drugs, especially crack and to engage in unprotected sex during hustling. He also refused any suggestions regarding drug treatment. His parting shot always was, "Don't worry, I can handle it. I can stop it."

I had naively thought that the combination of the good test results regarding Carlos' health status, the new information he had regarding his infection and ways he could actively maintain his health would be enough to help motivate him to seek drug treatment. My initial empathic and nonjudgmental stance had helped me to form a trusting relationship with him, but it also enabled Carlos to continue his drugging and hustling. Another style of intervention would now be needed if Carlos was ever going to go into drug treatment. It was suddenly very clear that Carlos' HIV infection was not his problem. In fact, it was much more likely that he would die from a drug overdose or some consequence of drug behavior than any HIV related illness.

I decided that from this point on my work with Carlos must focus on overcoming his denial and confronting his self-destructive behavior. All the other treatment goals I had developed to help him learn to live with HIV, e.g., explore his sexual identity, go back to school, or enter a job training program would have to take a back seat to the central problem in his life—his addiction. In any event, these other issues could be not worked through until Carlos was off drugs and sober.

I recognized that the adolescent AIDS program and the people in it were the only support system Carlos had in his life. While the interventions needed to be firm and consistent if they were to be successful, they could not be too demanding or strident, or he would not return to the program and receive his necessary medical care. I also knew this new strategy of working with Carlos needed to be supported and carried out by the entire treatment team. As a team, then, we developed the following treatment plan for Carlos: all team members, including the doctors, nurses, health educators and myself would, whenever possible, relate Carlos' health concerns and symptoms to his primary disease of drug addiction and not to his HIV infection; provide Carlos with drug education based on the disease model of addiction; and give him the message that he could not deal with his addiction alone, but that he needed the help of a drug treatment program.

Over the next couple of months, Carlos would sporadically appear in the clinic complaining of wheezing in his chest or a continuing weight loss. Each time his doctor would explain that Carlos' continued crack smoking was aggravating his chronic asthma and promoting his weight loss. Each member of the team patiently explained to him, time and again, that while pneumonia and weight loss were associated with advanced HIV disease, his symptoms were due solely to crack.

After each medical appointment, Carlos would stop in to see me. At these times he often appeared to be sad and contrite. He was beginning to see that crack was destroying his life. Yet, as soon as I mentioned drug treatment, he'd go back into denial and tell me he'd stop without treatment. When I inquired why he was so against treatment, he replied, "I don't want to be sent away again." I informed him about several outpatient day programs and explained that drug treatment did not mean, necessarily, that he would be sent away. However, Carlos continued to refuse to go into any kind of drug treatment. I confronted his assertion that "I can do it by myself" with "then do it." I asked Carlos if he could stay away from crack for one week. He said he could. We agreed to test this out, and I made an appointment with him for the following week to see how he was doing in his attempt to stop crack on his own.

I wasn't surprised when I didn't see Carlos for the next few weeks. When he did come in, he had a sexually transmitted disease (STD). After he was treated, he stopped by my office as usual. He told me he had an STD. I wondered aloud how difficult it must be to remember to use condoms when you are "high." Carlos told me he always used condoms, but that sometimes they break. This was the first time I knew he was lying to me. I predicted that if he continued to use crack and the other drugs, he'd continue to get STDS, lose weight, and get sick. I reminded him that his immune system was still in good shape, but that he wasn't doing anything to keep it that way, in fact, he was destroying his immune system. I realized I had just given another lecture that would have about the same effect all my others had. I became quiet and felt very angry and frustrated. Finally, after some moments of silence, I asked Carlos if he wanted to die. He suddenly looked defeated and said no. For the first time there was a hint of tears in his eyes. He said if I could find him a drug treatment program where he didn't have to go away from home, he would go.

I found a drug treatment program with both inpatient and outpatient components that agreed to interview Carlos. Carlos showed up for the appointment on time accompanied by his grandmother. He was first seen by the intake worker and then the director of the outpatient program. The director told us he could not accept Carlos for outpatient day treatment because he felt that both the severity and length of Carlos' drug addiction combined with the drug infested neighborhood Carlos lived in would jeopardize any hope of treatment success. The director recommended placement with their 18 month inpatient program and made an appointment with the inpatient department for Carlos the following week.

Carlos was disappointed and angry about the decision. He complained again that he didn't want to go away for inpatient treatment. Carlos' grandmother told him she also didn't want him to go away. As I pushed him to consider keeping his appointment with the inpatient program, Carlos angrily replied, "I don't want to waste eighteen months of what I got left in drug treatment." Carlos did not make the second appointment and disappeared from view for the next few weeks.

The next time I heard from Carlos he had been picked up by the police for drug possession. He called me from jail and asked me if I would come and visit him. During the visit, Carlos said, "In a way I'm glad I'm here, and I never thought I'd say that, but if I stayed on the streets any longer I'd be dead." Later, I was able to get Carlos transferred to a drug treatment within the jail. Because he had violated his probation he was not eligible for release, but there was a possibility he could serve out his sentence in a long term drug treatment center if he was motivated and did well in the prison based drug program. In the past few weeks, I've heard Carlos is doing well in the prison based drug program and is waiting on the judge's decision whether he can enter long-term residential drug treatment in lieu of a prison sentence.

The case example illustrates the need for the worker to first address the chemically dependent, HIV positive adolescent's substance abuse before attempting to help the adolescent work through the expected medical and psychosocial tasks that are associated with HIV disease. The intervention just described seemed to be the treatment strategy that was best able to confront this adolescent's strong denial system and motivate the client to ultimately accept drug and alcohol treatment. The intervention consisted of three stages: (1) assessment, (2) education and motivation to seek chemical dependency treatment and (3) referral and placement into appropriate treatment.

The first stage in the process depends on the taking of a careful and extensive substance use history. This history-taking can be a part of the general psychosocial history. The following substance use inventory is suggested: (1) frequency and quantity of each substance used, (2) patterns of use, abuse, and dependency of each substance over time, (3) setting in which each substance is used, (4) behaviors associated with use, abuse, and dependency, (5) peer involvement, (6) how substances are obtained and (7) the impact of use, abuse and dependency on family, friends, school, job, and the criminal justice system. The assessment should be viewed as on ongoing process. As the adolescent establishes a trusting relationship with the worker, additional information often emerges.

The second stage relies on the information gathered during the first stage. The history taking process itself is often the first time the adolescent acknowledges the extent and nature of her or his chemical dependency. In the education and motivation stage, the worker uses this knowledge of the adolescent's substance abuse and the self-destructive behavior that results from it to confront the adolescent with the consequences of their chemical dependency. The denial system of the particular adolescent is often so strong that the worker will have to confront this issue again and again over time. As a part of the ongoing confrontation, the worker can begin to predict future negative consequences that are particular to and appropriate for that adolescent.

During this stage, it is also important to enlist the help of family, friends and significant others (when possible) to present a united front in confronting the adolescent's denial. For many disenfranchised HIV positive adolescents, certain agency staff often function as surrogate family and these staff members, therefore, must be included in the intervention process. The work to motivate chemically dependent adolescents to seek treatment is often frustrating and time consuming. It is important for the worker to acknowledge that it is developmentally appropriate for the adolescent to initially reject the dependency and regression that is involved in chemical dependency treatment. Most adolescents feel they are invulnerable and can help themselves without adult supervision. Here, the worker must help the adolescent understand that no one can fight chemical dependency without the support of appropriate treatment.

Once the adolescent has made a commitment to enter treatment, the worker must be able to move quickly to place the adolescent in a treatment program that has the best chance of treating that particular adolescent's chemical dependency. In my experience, the adolescent's commitment is often time-limited and tends to revert to denial and resistance as the adolescent returns to his substance abuse and abusing family and/or peer group. During the time between the adolescent's decision to enter treatment and the intake appointment, the worker may need to provide additional time and support to the client.

To ensure rapid placement in a treatment program, the worker can develop and maintain a referral list of the various drug and alcohol treatment programs that are appropriate for adolescents. The list should contain the following information that is specific for HIV positive adolescents: (1) does the program accept HIV positive persons, (2) are HIV positive adolescents presently in the program, (3) has the staff been trained to work with HIV positive people, (4) does the program provide HIV medical and psychosocial treatment along with chemical dependency treatment, and (5) what is the program's policy regarding confidentiality and HIV. Additional information regarding the nature and philosophy of treatment, admission requirements, and financial arrangements is also important. The worker's familiarity with the treatment program and its staff can help calm the adolescent's fears during the waiting period prior to admission. I recommend that the worker accompany the adolescent to the intake meeting and also on admission. Many HIV positive chemically dependent adolescents do not have the support system that is necessary to sustain them during this part of the placement process. The intervention can be considered successful and completed when the adolescent is placed in the program.

Successful interventions with HIV positive chemically dependent adolescents are often frustrating and difficult for the worker involved. However, there is really no alternative to chemical dependency treatment. For many of the adolescents their treatment and twelve-step groups give their life new meaning. Sobriety for the adolescent and the support system that comes with it can also prove to be an incalculable benefit in meeting the challenges of living and thriving with HIV disease.

REFERENCES

Bell, T. and Hein, K. (1984). "The adolescent and sexually transmitted diseases." In K. Holmes, (Ed.) *Sexually Transmitted Diseases*. New York: Mc-Graw-Hill, 73-84.

Drucker, E. (1986). "AIDS and addiction in New York City" *American Journal of Alcohol and Drug Abuse*. 12(1/2), 165-181.

Fullilove, M. and Fullilove, R. (1989). "Intersecting epidemics: black teen crack use and sexually transmitted disease" *Journal of American Medical Women's Association*. 48(5), 146-153.

Futterman, D. (1990). "Medical management of adolescents" in *pediatric AIDS: the challenge of HIV infection in infants, children and adolescents*. In P. Pizzo & C. Wilfert, (Eds.) Baltimore: Williams and Wilkins, 546-560.

Futterman, D., Hein, K., Kipke, M., Reulbach, W., et al. (1990). "HIV and adolescents: HIV testing experiences and changes in Risk-Related Sexual and Drug Behavior." Presented at Sixth International Conference on AIDS.

Futterman, D., Reuben, N. and Hein, K. (1990). "HIV infection and adolescents: risk behaviors and models of care." Presented at Society of Adolescent Medicine.

Hein, K., (1989). "Commentary on adolescent Acquired Immunodeficiency Syndrome: the next wave of the Human Immunodeficiency Virus epidemic?" *The Journal of Pediatrics*, 114(1)., 144-149.

Hein, K., (1990). "Lessons from New York City on HIV/AIDS in adolescents." *New York State Journal of Medicine*, 90(3), 143-145.

Morehouse, E. (1989). "Treating adolescent alcohol abusers." *Social Casework*, 70(6), 355-363.

Quinn, T.C., Glasser, D., Stricof, R. et al. (1988). "Human Immunodeficiency

Virus infection among patients attending clinics for sexually transmitted diseases." *New England Journal of Medicine*. 318(4), 197-203.

Remafedi, G. (1988). "Preventing the sexual transmission of AIDS during adolescence." *Journal of Adolescent Health Care*. 9(2), 139-143.

St. Louis, M. Hayman, C. and Miller, C. (1989). "HIV infection in disadvantaged adolescents in the United States." Presented at Fifth International AIDS Conference.

Stiffman, A. and Earls, F. (1990). "Behavioral risk for HIV infection in adolescent medical patients." *Pediatrics* 85(3), 303-310.

Vermund, S.H., Hein, K., Gayle, H.D. et al. (1988). "Adolescent AIDS in New York City: predominance of central and drug related transmission." Presented at the Fourth International Conference on AIDS.

Working with Chemically Dependent HIV Infected Patients on an Inpatient Medical Unit

Carol J. Weiss, MD

Working with the chemically dependent HIV infected patient on an inpatient medical unit poses special problems for the medical staff. These patients are perceived as irresponsible, manipulative, demanding, drug-seeking trouble makers. They rarely follow the rules of the ward, such as not smoking, not leaving the floor, and not using drugs. Staff often feel violated and abused by these patients.

Medical and nursing staff working with these patients need support and education to help them with this population. To achieve this, support groups, didactic lectures, management seminars, and consultation on individual patients can be provided by someone with expertise in chemical dependency. This consultant can also be present at meetings addressing policy issues such as illicit drug use on the unit and discharge against medical advice.

Staff working with this population needs to change their level of expectation regarding these patients. For example, compliance in this population is not the same as in other populations. These patients may not be accustomed to taking medications regularly or arriving reliably for all appointments. These patients may comply erratically at first, improving their compliance as they become more acclimated to the regimen or develop more trust in the medication and/or hospital. This process may take weeks to years.

Patients do not necessarily change their behavior just because they've entered a hospital. A person who is accustomed to getting his/her drugs when she/he wants it, may have difficulty waiting for medication or declining the drugs offered by visiting guests. When staff feels less offended and angered by this behavior, they may be better able to work with this population.

Unless the medical unit is equipped to search patients' possessions and rooms regularly and restrict visitors, illicit drug use on the ward is unavoidable. Once staff understands this, their efforts can be directed towards minimizing this phenomenon and its consequences. They can attempt to ensure that the patient is adequately medicated with licit drugs; they can obtain urine toxicology to determine which patients are engaging in such behavior; they can target patients who are using illicit drugs on the unit and either restrict their visitors or post a companion to observe them.

The drug dependent patient usually requires generous amounts of medication while in the hospital. Staff often withhold from these patients the very medication they need, making these patients even more irritable and difficult to manage. Making the patient comfortable with adequate opiates or sedatives will help the patient feel heard; it will enhance the patient's trust and improve the working relationship between the chemically dependent patient and medical or nursing staff.

Once such a trust is established, it is easier for the patient to accept the limits that staff will need to place, such as frequent urine toxicologies and occasional room searches or visitor restriction. These limits should be set respectfully but without embarrassment. The patient should be advised that these are necessary, sensible precautions that are instituted for all patients with chemical dependency problems. It is not an indictment against any particular patient or an indication that any particular patient is not trusted. It is merely a safeguard to help the patient deal with the common and understandable problem of drug use on the unit.

The following case vignettes illustrate two ways of managing a chemically dependent medical inpatient.

CASE 1

Mr. R, an HIV positive intravenous drug user, was admitted to the hospital with suspected pneumonia. He begins to ask for pain medication immediately upon admission. The nurses distaste for this patient is apparent. He calls for nursing many times during the four hours he waits to see the doctor. The doctor agrees to give him Percodan for pain. Over the next two days, the patient is demanding and irritable, calling the nurses frequently, complaining of physical discomfort and asking for pain medication or Valium. The nurses begin to ignore the patient's calls, which leads him to begin screaming demands and shouting obscenities. After Mr. R's wife comes to visit him, he is calm and sedated. Staff strongly suspect Mr. R used drugs brought to him by his wife. They feel violated and abused by Mr. R and wish he could be asked to leave the hospital. Mr. R signs out against medical advice on the third day after being admitted.

CASE 2

Mr. H is also an HIV positive intravenous drug user and was admitted to the hospital with diarrhea. On admission, he immediately begins to demand "something to calm me down." Nursing staff establishes that he injects four to six bags of heroin a day and has not injected any in almost twenty-four hours. They inform the patient that they understand that he is in withdrawal and will attempt to notify the physician to receive orders for methadone as soon as possible. They also inform the patient that they will need to obtain a urine drug toxicology test, which is standard procedure for all their chemically dependent patients, and may also be taking urine tests 2-3 times a week while he is in the hospital. The nurses explain that this too is standard procedure and is for the patient's protection as well as staff's.

Mr. H waits two hours to receive 20 mg of methadone. Two hours later, he complains that he needs more medication and is given another 10 mg. The following day, Mr. H is quiet until 3 p.m. when he begins to ring frequently for the nurses. Because he is demanding more medication, he is seen by the substance abuse consultant who learns that he dropped out of his methadone program three months ago. He had been maintained there for years on 80 mgs of methadone. A phone call to the program confirms this.

Mr. H's methadone dose is increased over the next two days to 60 mg., at which point the patient ceases to complain of discomfort.

Sometimes, chemically dependent patients may be demanding even after they have received adequate medication. In this case, they may not be demanding medication, but services such as cigarettes or a blanket. If their requests of staff become excessive, this should be addressed directly, not ignored and silently resented. The patient should be firmly told that you would like to be of as much help as possible, but you are busy with many patients and the patient must understand that and be patient. This respectful expression of concern and limit setting will be perceived much more favorably by the patient than resentment and avoidance.

Hospital staff usually do not have the time or training to provide drug treatment for these patients. Staff should understand that this is best accomplished *after* the medical hospitalization when the patient can be referred to a comprehensive treatment program. The role of the hospital staff is to help the patient be comfortable so that she/he may receive adequate medical care, not to provide drug rehabilitation treatment.

The substance abuse consultant can work with the patient to determine the appropriate treatment program. Some patients can be transferred directly to rehabilitation programs. Appointments for intake interviews should be made while the patient is in the hospital. Some hospitals have Twelve-Step program meetings on the premises which patients may attend. Delegates from various twelve-step groups are sometimes available to visit hospitalized patients. A support group for hospitalized chemically dependent patients can also be organized to help motivate and inform patients.

Slow detoxification from sedatives may also occur in the hospital setting during concurrent medical treatment. Opiate detoxification is advised in instances where the patient may be transferred to a therapeutic community. Otherwise, methadone maintenance is the preferred treatment for illicit opiate dependence in this population.

Sometimes hospitalized patients on methadone maintenance request rapid detoxification from methadone while in the hospital. This is ill-advised as relapse to opiate use is highly likely in this setting. Slow detoxification in the setting of extensive therapeutic support — usually outpatient — is much preferred. If the patient insists on rapid detoxification, their need for immediate gratification should be addressed.

The work of hospital staff is often made more difficult by certain common assumptions made about HIV infected chemically dependent patients. Staff may feel that it is a futile effort to rehabilitate these patients, or they may believe that chemically dependent patients just do not want to stop taking drugs. After all, the fact that they are still using attests to that.

Staff may assume that using drugs or alcohol is pleasurable and that people addicted to these substances are enjoying themselves. Their belief about HIV infected people is that they're going to die anyway, so why take away their pleasure? Why not let them enjoy the final years?

Another common assumption is that chemically dependent people with HIV disease lack the motivation necessary for recovery. Getting off drugs or alcohol requires such hard work; why would someone with HIV disease burden themselves with such a struggle? Also, people kick drugs to live a better life. Why work for a better life if you have a fatal disease?

In response to such assumptions, it is important to understand that most addicts have stopped enjoying intoxication for quite a while. For some people, an occasional drink may be enjoyable, but for the addict, substance use is rarely pleasurable; for them, it is a dread compulsion and a guaranteed continuation of their depression, demoralization, and chaotic lifestyle.

Most addicts want to quit and have tried to do so many times. They usually have felt much better about themselves and much more hopeful about the world when they have been clean. It would be pleasurable for them to be clean and not live with the high price of addiction; demoralization, impairment in health, loss of money, and sometimes loss of home and loved ones. The chemically dependent person with HIV disease usually wants to enjoy the remainder of his or her life and is in a much better position to do so off drugs and alcohol.

Not all people with life threatening illnesses give up on life. Chemically dependent patients, like all patients, have a variety of responses to their illness, and these responses change over the course of the years they live with their diagnosis. Fear and fatalism may be an early response. During this phase, chemically dependent patients who actively use illicit drugs may use their familiar and historic coping mechanism, often to excess. Some patients in recovery relapse during this period. However, hope and lust for life is also a response experienced by chemically dependent patients and this can be a powerful motivator for recovery.

CASE 3

Mr. B is a 26 year old HIV positive intravenous drug user. He has known of his HIV status for nine months. He was a resident at a therapeutic community for eighteen months and dropped out three months after learning his serostatus. At first, after dropping out, he attended Narcotics Anonymous meetings, and was drug free, but relapsed to intravenous drug use within a month. For the past five months, he has been using drugs and living with his mother who occasionally kicks him out of the house.

On the unit, Mr. B. is unkempt and does not look up when spoken to. He appears either irritable or sedated most of the time. When approached about chemical dependency treatment, he says, "What's the use? I'm going to die anyway." In working with him, the chemical dependency consultant points out that HIV is not a death sentence. It is pointed out to him that he has many more years to live, especially if he lives drug free. Examples of other HIV positive patients who have undergone chemical dependency treatment and gone on to enjoy their lives and families are presented to him.

Mr. B continues to decline referral to treatment for seven days. On the eighth day, he begins to read some Twelve-Step literature he has brought with him into the hospital. He requests that friends from treatment visit him. After discharge, Mr. B begins to attend an outpatient drug rehabilitation program and daily NA meetings.

The fact that a patient continues to use substances is not evidence that they don't want to quit. Getting off drugs and alcohol is not an issue of will; it is an issue of being in appropriate treatment. Treatment works and most people will quit when placed in appropriate treatment. Sometimes people remain abstinent for months, sometimes years, and sometimes forever. Sometimes people require multiple treatments to get better. But the main point to remember is that treatment works and people require treatment, not will, to stop abusing substances.

Some patients resist treatment. This does not necessarily mean that they don't want to stop using substances. They usually resist for other reasons, namely pride, shame, fear, and demoralization. For example, they're too proud to ask for help. They insist on trying to stop by themselves; this usually leads to failure. After multiple failures, they may become ashamed and do not want to expose their failures to others. They may say, "I didn't want to quit anyway." Fear of life without familiar substances and fear of failure also contribute to treatment refusal. Finally, the weight of demoralization keeps people entrenched in behaviors they might wish to change were they to have the energy and spirit to do so.

Another source of resistance is wishful or magical thinking. Some patients have the idea that now that they are medically ill and realize how precious life is, they would not think of using drugs any more. This denial, or naivete, about the tenacity of a lifelong style of coping is quite common and can be addressed without wounding the patient's pride.

The following is a prototypic exchange with such a patient:

> Staff: "I feel you should get involved in a chemical dependency treatment program after discharge from the hospital."
>
> Patient: "Thanks for your help, but I don't need one of those programs. I know I'm never going to use again. I can't. I just came this close to dying and I know now I want to live. Believe me, I want to live. When I want something this bad, I don't need help; I'm not going to need a drug treatment program."
>
> Staff: "I believe you that you don't want to use anymore, and I believe you that you don't plan to use anymore. You mean it with all your heart, and I know that. I trust you that you are

being sincere with me. But I know from experience that it takes more than will or desire or intent to stop using drugs. It is not so easy to quit and stay quit. Don't tell me you don't know that, otherwise you would have been clean a long time already. It takes help.''

"You've been using drugs for many years. You've used drugs when you're lonely, when you're with friends, when you're angry, when you want to celebrate, when you're sad, when you're scared, when you're bored, or for no reason at all, just out of habit. This way of dealing with life doesn't just go away. It took you years to learn to use drugs and make them a part of your life; it will take time for you to learn to not use drugs. You need a whole new education on how to live clean, and that takes time. You can't assume it will come naturally.''

"And you don't just get things because you want it, and you don't get it overnight. That's unrealistic; that's a junkie's mentality. You've got to work for this goal and go to school for this goal, and that's what treatment is.''

Patient: "I don't have the time. I've got things to do. I've got AIDS, and I need to be with my family.''

Staff: "Your family would be much happier to see you in treatment. As a matter of fact, I can't think of anything that would make them happier than to see you in treatment. You'll be much better off and better for your family if you do it.''

Engaging the resistent chemically dependent patient entails discerning their particular resistance and finding that part within them that wants to address their addiction. Some patients cannot be reached, but they are the minority. These patients are best left alone so that providers' energy can be used with others.

Each patient has their own idiosyncratic fears about treatment. The substance abuse consultant, who is familiar with these different fears, can meet a few times with the patient to help delineate what these fears are. Sometimes people have bad associations with a friend or neighbor who went into treatment. Some people have the belief that entering treatment confirms that they are a failure, especially if they have already been through treatment in the past. Others fear they'll be brainwashed or ridiculed. Once these fears are expressed and labelled, the active drug user is usually more amenable to intervention. Patients can be shown that seeking help is a sign of strength, not weakness. Or they can be told that some people require going through treatment many times before it finally takes hold.

In an ideal world, drug treatment could be provided on site during medical hospitalization. For many reasons, the medical hospital is ideally suited for this role:

1. There is a high concentration of chemically dependent patients in the hospital.
2. Hospitalization is an auspicious time when these patients are stationery, vulnerable, and accessible for days to weeks, making repeated and sustained interventions possible.
3. Acute medical illness and hospitalization are often times when chemically dependent patients are highly motivated to cease drug use and follow through with referral efforts.
4. During hospitalization, these patients are usually unoccupied, bored, and profoundly anxious; they are often desperately looking for something to do, especially therapeutic contact.

The medical unit could have regular chemical dependency groups, educational seminars, family meetings, and individual counseling, twelve-step meetings as well as medical treatment. Unfortunately, such a unit does not yet exist. For now, given the dearth of such innovative programs, the best treatment that can be provided for chemically dependent HIV infected patients remains intelligent assessment and referral, rational day-to-day management, and compassion.

Short Term Group Work with Intravenous Drug Using People with AIDS in a Hospital Setting

Paul A. Zakrzewski, MSW

The profile of intravenous drug using patients — a profile of isolated, disenfranchised, and misunderstood people — has implications far surpassing those for any other group at high risk for contracting AIDS (Caputo, 1985). This article reports on one model for helping the health care worker in a hospital setting provide much needed psycho-social support to hospitalized intravenous drug using individuals who are symptomatic with HIV illness.

GROUP WORK FOR IVDUs IN THE HOSPITAL SETTING

Group work has proved to be a powerful modality in the treatment of gay men with AIDS. It is clear that a diagnosis of AIDS touches off many similar emotional reactions in IVDUs as in gay men. Diagnosis adds to both groups of patients' sadness, depression, and burden of unresolved grief (Gambe & Getzel, 1989). But there the similarity ends. A diagnosis of AIDS often triggers a cynical, almost apathetic reaction in an IVDU. He/she may see it as just another lousy hand which life or the system has dealt him/her. Therefore the need for group work with this population is critical. In 1987 the author and a coleader began an inpatient group for IVDUs with AIDS at Bellevue Hospital in Manhattan.

55

FORMATION AND DEVELOPMENT

The first question that needed to be addressed was the efficacy of having both gay men and IVDUs in the same group. We discovered that an AIDS support group comprised of both gays and IVDU's was counterproductive to the aims of mutual support and mutual aid. While both populations shared the experience of having a diagnosis of AIDS, the disparities in lifestyle often created barriers to group homogeneity. Support comes partly from a feeling of commonality, the "we're in the same boat, brother" theme, the dynamic change mechanism of universality. During the first session, Jorge a twenty-four year-old Latino male who grew up in the Bronx and was currently at Rikers Island serving a sentence for armed robbery stated openly, "I have no respect for faggots. I seen them in prison always coming on to you. I'd as soon bust one in the mouth as look at 'em." In response David, a 37 year-old white gay designer from Cleveland said, "It's scum like you that make me sick. You probably mugged old ladies to buy your drugs." While one might argue that such an interaction might open up a group exploration related to the issues of racism, classism, and homophobia, that was not the objective of this particular group. All this interaction served to do was to create tension between the two groups and obscure the real issues confronting an IVDU with AIDS. As a result, both groups stayed away from the group.

It was clear that there were many groups in place for gay men with AIDS within the community. The hospitalized IVDUs needed a group geared to the specific issues confronting them. There is little sense of community among drug abusers, even when there are common threads such as color, ethnicity, and an AIDS diagnosis. An attempt to form a group was a difficult, but not impossible task for the social worker (Caputo, 1985). The support and assistance they gained through group interaction led to solutions and a feeling of self-empowerment.

My experience has been that when working with this population in a hospital setting the group worked best when it was time-limited, running either eight or ten sessions. The fact that a long commitment was not required helped make the group seem viable to potential members. Attendance was purely voluntary. When a patient was discharged from the hospital during the ten-week cycle, arrangements were made for the member to continue attending until the ten week cycle was completed. When group members wished to continue in a group after the initial ten weeks were over, another ongoing, weekly group was provided. Group size was limited to ten members, and included both men and women.

These groups were co-led by a social worker and a nurse/AIDS health educator. Having two leaders who had overlapping areas of expertise and who were able to support one another during the group was essential. Both of the co-leaders had solid clinical backgrounds in chemical dependency which was also essential in working with this population. Potential group members were screened individually by both group leaders. The criteria for inclusion were a diagnosis of AIDS, a history of alcohol or drug abuse or dependency, a commitment to abstinence from all chemicals, and a willingness to participate in the entire ten-week process. Individual interviews were useful in understanding and clarifying the particular goals that clients hoped to achieve and their reactions to the available services and the conditions under which the help was given, (Northen, 1988).

The psychological-clinical approach might have some validity in working with patients who were domiciled, employed, and connected to support systems. But with a patient population of people with AIDS, (PWAs), who were IVDUs a different approach was required. The emphasis needed to be on education and acculturation to the hospital care system if their needs were to be addressed and met.

During the interviews with potential group members the issues they reported as primary had to do with being homeless; without funds, food, social support systems, and medical coverage; frustration at what they perceived as hostility on the part of medical and nursing staff; chemical dependency; and finally AIDS. Thus themes that the group needed to address included such questions as: How can an IVDU who is newly diagnosed with AIDS focus on issues related to illness, death and dying when his/her basic survival needs aren't being met? How does an IVDU break out of his/her cycle of denial and isolation to seek help by attending a group? How can issues related to substance abuse be addressed? How can patients learn to communicate their needs to medical, nursing, and social service staff in less hostile, demanding, and threatening ways? An ongoing difficulty in running this group was helping group members deal with the critical illness or death of group members over time.

GROUP OBJECTIVES

Facilitating groups for hospitalized IVDUs with AIDS over the last three years has led me to develop specific group goals. Hospitalized IVDUs with AIDS need: (1) to explore ways to communicate clearly and appropriately with the treatment team to gain a clarity and understanding of their diagnosis and their treatment plan so that they may participate in treatment more fully; (2) to understand entitlement related to shelter, food, and medical treatment; (3) to understand how their substance abuse impacts on the development of HIV infection; (4) to explore ways to support each other in remaining abstinent and sober; (5) to develop an after-care plan which supports abstinence and sobriety upon discharge; (6) to freely express and share their feelings of sadness, fear, anger, and uncertainty related to a diagnosis of AIDS, as well as feelings about death and dying; (7) to share positive ways each member copes with the illness; (8) to participate in activities that reinforce a positive outlook and hope; (9) to develop ways to retain control of their lives while in the hospital; (10) to express gratitude to those staff members who are caring.

PHASES OF GROUP DEVELOPMENT

The groups usually had four distinct phases. The first was a testing-out situation in which directly expressed hostility toward the hospital created group unity. The second phase was characterized by the expression of anxiety-laden fantasies. The third phase occurred when feelings towards one another began to be shared and introspective thinking was possible. The fourth and closing phase occurred when members began to focus on the outside world and make plans for what they would do when they left the institution.

The first phase of the group was a period of education and orientation that lasted from four to five sessions. An important aspect of this phase was the hostility and rage group members expressed towards members of the medical staff. During this period members were encouraged to ask questions about AIDS, the various opportunistic infections which they might have, its transmission, and prevention. Safer sex and safer needle use were repeatedly stressed. During this phase financial and housing entitlement were clarified. In addition, issues surrounding their drug use and dependency began to be revealed. It was essential that one of the leaders had an understanding of chemical dependency and the available treatment options and resources.

Before a patient was interviewed for group membership, the workers checked each patient's chart and consulted with the patient's social worker to make certain that the patient had a diagnosis of AIDS. Many patients were confused by their diagnoses. It is worth mentioning that even though the members have been told the group is for persons with AIDS few members mentioned their diagnosis when introducing themselves to the group members. They often denied they had AIDS by identifying their illness by the name of their opportunistic infection.

When Rose, a 28 year-old black prostitute arrived for the first session she stated, "I guess I don't belong in the group. I don't have AIDS." The nurse/health educator explored this further with Rose in the group. Rose said that the original intern told her she had AIDS but that he must have made a mistake because the new intern told her that she no longer had AIDS. When the worker questioned Rose further, it was revealed that the doctor told Rose that she had disseminated TB, which Rose took to mean she didn't have AIDS. The nurse/health educator gave Rose the information she needed to understand her diagnosis. Other group members expressed things they were confused about related to their diagnosis and by the end of the session there was a level of clarity about AIDS and diagnoses. Those patients who were still confused were referred back to their doctors with an understanding of how to approach the doctors in order to have their confusion resolved.

The second part of this phase relates to patient-staff relations and the patients' rage about it. The group members recounted stories of staff members' neglect and lack of respect towards them. A prolonged hospital stay not only produces stress in the patient, it also has a profoundly negative effect on the staff especially in those cases where there is friction between staff and patients.

During the session in which staff relations were addressed, it was helpful that a member of the medical/nursing staff was present. This arrangement indicated to the group members that staff was concerned about their issues and complaints, and it provided a buffer against the indifference of abusive staff members.

Jorge, a 24 year-old Hispanic IVDU was hospitalized in order to receive chemotherapy for Burketts Lymphoma. He discussed a situation in which the abdominal pain became so intense that he requested pain medication. He described screaming and demanding medication to decrease the pain. The intern who was assigned to his case refused medication. In the process, Jorge became more demanding and verbally abusive. The intern responded by calling Jorge a "junkie liar" and again refused to order pain medication on the grounds he was simply looking for a quick fix.

The nursing staff on duty while this incident occurred were so distressed by the young doctor's behavior that they phoned for the resident and a consulting doctor on the AIDS Team. The AIDS Team's doctor recommended that Jorge be given the pain medication immediately, to which the resident responded, "He's faking, and I refuse to be manipulated." At this point, Jorge lost control and lunged at the young doctor who called the hospital police who arrested Jorge and had him shackled to his bed for the remainder of his hospital stay.

When hearing the story described above, the leaders empathized with Jorge and began to problem solve with the group about how similar situations could be prevented in the future. This situation was explored by the worker role playing the part of Jorge while Jorge role played the young doctor. Jorge was able to reach inside himself and express thoughts and feelings which may have been going on inside of the doctor related to being overworked, unappreciated, and threatened by patients on a daily basis. The group began to listen and coach the worker from the sideline as to how to modify his behavior in an attempt to get his needs met. Members began to verbalize insight into how their own attitudes were adding to the tension between them and the staff. They began to understand how the system operates and what the medical and nursing staff are up against in delivering services to them.

An initial challenge for the leaders had been how to recruit members for such a group when staff attitudes towards it were negative and often hostile. However, three weeks after the group began the head nurse on the unit to which Jorge was assigned contacted the co-leaders to inform them, "I don't know what you're telling that boy, but he has sure turned his attitude around." We asked her to mention this to Jorge directly in order to help him understand the positive consequences of his new behavior with staff. This kind of change was the best publicity for getting new referrals to the group and led to the development of alliances between staff and patients within the group.

The onset of the second phase of the group was characterized by many members expressing a belief that AIDS and the availability of drugs in minority communities were conspiracies on the part of the white establishment to eliminate minorities. This is best exemplified by the case of Peter who is a 33 year-old black male with a diagnosis of AIDS. Prior to being hospitalized he had been living in a shooting gallery. Peter is a crack abuser with a long history of heroin IV use. At the beginning of one session, he began passing around an article in which the CIA was cited as the having developed HIV to rid the world of all undesirable such as gays, drug users, Blacks, and Hispanics. Peter became enraged and started vilifying the government and threatening to assassinate as many as he could when released from the hospital. He stated he didn't care how many lives he took as long as he got revenge for the horrendous plot perpetrated against him. Other members of the group joined in with their own tales of plots against Blacks or Hispanics.

For the next two sessions every discussion led back to the discussion of a plot. Hank, a 43 year-old white male, who was recently released from the prison on a manslaughter charge, discussed the rage he felt at his girlfriend for dumping him after she heard he had been diagnosed with AIDS. He said he fantasized about going back to her apartment and taking a knife and stabbing himself and bleeding all over his girlfriend. "Maybe she'll get AIDS and know how lonely and fearful it feels." At that point Peter broke down sobbing. He admitted to being frightened about his diagnosis and what was going to happen to him when he was discharged from the hospital. His mother and his wife refused to let him live with them. He said, "They're just like the CIA; they'd be happy to see me dead." This opened up an opportunity for the female worker to role play the part of Peter's mother and wife in which she expressed fear of the disease and anger at Peter's continued drug use. To this Peter replied, "Why the fuck shouldn't I keep using drugs. I'm thinking that if things get too bad, I'll just kill myself by overdosing. This way I choose the time."

This opened the way for a discussion about treatment options for HIV infection which many IVDUs see as mechanisms by which the government can use them as "guinea pigs" and possibly infect them further. This was an opportunity for the workers to explore the reality of these fears with the group members as well as the effects of illegal drugs on the immune system and the benefits of abstaining from drug and alcohol use. Treatment options for their chemical dependency were presented and explored. There was little enthusiasm for giving up drugs, but as a result of this session, it was agreed that Alcoholics Anonymous (AA) and Narcotics Anonymous (NA) meetings would be initiated for patients with AIDS while in the hospital.

The third phase of the group began when members expressed less rage at the staff and were able to focus on themselves and the other group members. By sharing and listening, they begin to identify with one another, a process that helped them to accept and admit that they had a diagnosis of AIDS. The members began to rely on one another and looked forward to seeing each other every week. As the weeks progressed they expressed their appreciation for being able to see each other regularly and have a place to share feelings about the progression of their illness. The members began networking with one another, sharing information about AZT and other potential drug treatments. Members began to freely offer mutual aid and support as evidenced when a few members visited one another during the week.

During this phase the group members began to discuss more personal issues such as estrangement from children, family, wives, husbands, lovers, and friends. Discussions also centered around how to disclose one's diagnosis to family and friends.

Patricia a 35 year-old black woman discussed phoning her mother in Georgia to tell her about her diagnosis. She hoped for a reconciliation and an invitation to see her daughter whom she had abandoned to her mother. She admitted to the group that she had other motives. AIDS had awakened a need in her for care, support and a decent place in which to die. Her mother told Patricia that she got what she deserved; that God was punishing her. The mother refused to see her or to allow her to see her daughter. Rose finished by turning to the group and saying that she had burned all her bridges and this group was all she had that symbolized caring and support.

The fourth phase began when members began to express their hopes and fears. As they prepared to leave the hospital setting, they began to share their expectations about what awaited them. They vowed to abstain from using drugs or alcohol once they were discharged. They made plans despite the knowledge that any plans might have to be modified as their illness progressed.

After a few months in the hospital and attending group, patients had become much more realistic about the progression of AIDS. They had roommates who had died from or who had become physically and mentally incapacitated as a result of AIDS. While they resented being in the hospital, it provided a safety net as well as ongoing medical attention. Being discharged from the hospital was a mixed blessing and meant leaving the group which had been a source of support and aid.

Shortly after the first group began Robert, a 40 year-old black man, was discharged from the hospital. He was a very intelligent man who became addicted to heroin while serving in Vietnam. The group members knew that Robert was to be discharged, and no one expected him to show up for the group. When he arrived all members were surprised. Jorge made a sarcastic quip, ''What's the matter, you crazy to come back here once you out.'' Robert said that the group had become like a family to him and that he missed the support. He described the sleazy hotel to which he had been discharged as being filled with crack dealers and users. He was afraid if he didn't make contact with the group and attend his Narcotics Anonymous (NA) and Alcoholics Anonymous (AA) meetings he would just give up. "It's cold out there." That's all he kept repeating along with, "You're gonna see my face every week."

CONCLUSION

This model of short-term group work for IVDUs with AIDS within the hospital setting proved invaluable for both patient and staff alike. Due to the overwhelming staff shortage, groups of this kind can help reduce the strain on hospital staffs working with this often difficult to manage group of patients. In addition, the group interaction offers IVDUs the opportunity to think clearly about their substance abuse patterns if they are to be long-term survivors of HIV infection.

One of the most important outcomes of this group was that participants slowly began to view the doctors and nurses as allies rather than enemies, replacing the victim mentality with a sense of personal responsibility for the quality of their lives. As the weeks progressed, they got a clearer picture of how the rage they felt about the lack of control over their own lives spilled over into their interactions with the staff. The discussions began to center on self-empowerment. They were exploring the possibilities of what they might do to keep themselves occupied and positive while they were in the hospital.

If they wanted to stay off drugs, they had to take charge and go to NA meetings or treatment of some kind. This honesty about their drug problem made them look at who they were associating with in the hospital. They had to admit that if they started hanging around people who were dealing and using drugs they might not be able to resist the temptation. A few individuals did resume using drugs and stopped attending group. Yet the majority of people who elected to continue in the group did stay drug and alcohol free at least during their hospitalization. This was a major breakthrough. This model demonstrates that group work for hospitalized IVDUs with AIDS is able to serve the needs and address issues confronting these individuals during a time of extremely high stress.

REFERENCES

Caputo, L. (1985). "Dual diagnosis: AIDS and addiction. *Social Work*, 30(4), 361-364.

Gambe, R. and Getzel G. (1989). "Group work with gay men with AIDS." *Social Casework*, 70(3), 172-179.

Northen, H. (1988). *Social Work With Groups*. New York: Columbia University Press.

Persons with HIV
on Methadone Maintenance

Yvonne Harris, BA

The onset of AIDS/HIV disease has had an enormous impact on the clients and staff involved in methadone maintenance as a drug treatment modality. This article reports on some of the counseling issues that have arisen in a hospital based methadone maintenance treatment program located on the west side of Manhattan.

Methadone is the medication dispensed, not the treatment. The treatment is the process of seeing the people every day and providing psycho-social support for them. Effective treatment is composed of first forming a working relationship with people who are or who have been at the bottom-most rungs of our society. The staff must convey understanding, respect, commitment, as well as insight in order to develop a therapeutic alliance. Clients on methadone are different from and often more difficult to work with than even other chemically dependent clients. They have more social and health problems. Very often they have been using drugs intravenously for many years before beginning to take methadone. In many cases, they continue to use illicit drugs or drink alcoholically even when they are on methadone. Patients on methadone frequently are also struggling with issues of poverty, homelessness, crack, and AIDS. Many of our patients face all of these issues simultaneously on a daily basis. These are people who do not usually trust either the health care establishment or drug treatment professionals since most of the time they have not been treated with respect, care, or gentleness. The two cases presented below are typical of people with HIV illness who are on methadone.

Raul was a black male in his early fifties years who was a client of our methadone program for over eighteen years before his death in the late 1980s. He was admitted to the program in the early seventies when it functioned very much like a huge extended family. Prior to beginning methadone he had a long arrest history and spent most of his teenage and young adult life in prison as a result of drug related arrests. The years he was in the program he never was arrested or incarcerated. By replacing intravenous use of illicit heroin with methadone, he was soon able to obtain some stability in his previously erratic life. Even though Raul didn't finish high school, he could fix anything and enjoyed working with his hands. He eventually found employment as a handyman.

Going on methadone and stopping use of all other illicit drugs created a remarkable change in Raul who grew up a tough black kid in East Harlem, where he managed to survive through brute force which was the norm for many young men in that neighborhood. Prior to entering our program he had grown tired of a life defined by illegal activities and violence and wanted better for himself.

He had tried on many occasions to go into residential treatment programs but was always rejected due to his violent background. In an effort to stop using drugs, he had been medically detoxed from heroin five or six times as an inpatient but always relapsed shortly after being discharged.

Methadone provided Raul with the opportunity to stop the criminal activity and violence that had always been directly related to his heroin addiction. He eventually married, and after six years his wife died as a result of gynecological problems. For many years after her death, Raul lived alone. Growing tired of living alone and feeling lonely, he began to date. He soon met a woman named Bea with whom he began to spend all of his spare time. After Bea moved in with Raul, it soon became apparent that she had a serious drug problem.

Discussing this situation with his counselor, Raul came to accept that his own recovery would be in jeopardy if he continued to spend time with a woman who was using drugs. He decided to speak to Bea about going on methadone. Bea applied to and was accepted into our program.

Raul's problems were not solved with this intervention. Bea discontinued using heroin but discovered cocaine. Bea continued to use cocaine and participate in illicit behavior, thus creating a lot of problems in their relationship. She would often hang out with friends who were also using drugs, and he wouldn't see her for days. Finally he began to use cocaine himself.

It was not long before Raul's cocaine use had escalated to such a degree that he began to use his rent money to buy cocaine, resulting in their being evicted from his apartment. Raul moved in with a friend where Bea was not welcomed. This created obvious strains in their relationship. Raul's work performance was also suffering, and for the first time in years, his job was in jeopardy as a result of his drug use.

Finally he spoke to his counselor and asked for help with his cocaine problem. He was willing to be admitted to an inpatient detox. Raul really didn't want to break up with Bea, but the relationship had taken its toll on him. Raul became rather withdrawn and quite isolated as a result of the relationship with Bea ending.

Bea began to lose a lot of weight and was sick a lot of the time, with chronic respiratory problems in the form of bronchitis or pneumonia. In six months Bea had seven hospital admissions for one respiratory infection after another. While hospitalized, she would send messages to Raul asking him to visit her. He would never go but would send her money for cigarettes and for the television. In 1985 Bea was again hospitalized for pneumonia and died during this hospitalization. The unconfirmed rumors around the program were that she died of AIDS.

The same year that Bea died, Raul became part of an HIV research project at the clinic and tested positive for HIV antibodies. His denial about testing positive for HIV was so powerful that for three years he wouldn't discuss any feelings he had about having been exposed to HIV or that Bea might have died from AIDS. There was even a period of time when he denied ever having been involved with Bea. He refused any HIV monitoring or counseling. He asserted that nothing was wrong with him.

Raul's life remained stable following Bea's death, though he began to lose weight. The results of a required annual physical examination indicated problems. Though he never complained of any physical ailments, his blood chemistry began to show signs that he was immune compromised. Circulatory problems resulted in his legs swelling which made walking difficult. When he had been injecting drugs into the veins in his legs, he had had abscesses which had healed after he stopped shooting drugs. These began to become infected again after many years.

Raul's counselor attempted to discuss these various health concerns with him during sessions, yet Raul refused to admit that anything was wrong with him physically. When his counselor suggested that Raul might wish to attend health education programs at the clinic about HIV illness, Raul responded that he failed to see why the counselor continued to make this suggestion. Counseling sessions remained very superficial, with Raul only reporting on his life since the previous session.

Despite his deteriorating physical condition, Raul continued to work and come to the clinic regularly to pick up his methadone and get counseling. He would claim not to remember any information the doctors discussed with him regarding his HIV status. The counselor and the medical director of the clinic both were unable to determine whether this was symptomatic of HIV related dementia or just very powerful denial. He continued to grow weaker until he was unable to work, gave up his apartment, and moved in with his mother. When he became too weak to come into the clinic, a staff member would deliver a one-or two-week supply of methadone to him at home. Even during this time, Raul refused to acknowledge in discussions with his counselor any concerns about HIV or AIDS.

Raul also began to be hospitalized for various infections that would result in his remaining in the hospital for seven or eight weeks at a time. During one of these admissions, he was diagnosed as having toxoplasmosis and was placed on the AIDS unit. This was very helpful to Raul, as it finally broke through his denial about what was happening to his body. He felt more comfortable being on this unit than on a regular ward because everyone was equally sick. It was only after he was diagnosed with an AIDS related opportunistic infection that he began to talk about his fears and concerns pertaining to his having AIDS.

Raul vowed never to tell anyone that he had AIDS, not even his mother. His mother and clients from the program visited him in the hospital regularly. His friends from the methadone program all knew that Raul had AIDS but accepted his cues and acted like they didn't know what he was sick with. Raul's mother knew her son was very ill but had no idea that he had AIDS.

She found out he had AIDS when Raul was being discharged from his second hospitalization and the discharge clerk explained that Raul must return to be followed in the AIDS clinic. This was the first time Raul's mother had ever asked exactly what his illness was. Raul felt that after learning about his diagnosis his mother never treated him as well as she did prior to learning that he had AIDS. She was afraid to get close to him after that. She fed him on paper plates and gave him disposable plastic utensils. She was uncomfortable with his using the bathroom and prohibited him from using the kitchen at all. She herself used a portable toilet that was originally intended for him. He was excluded from all family activities and gatherings which no longer took place at his mother's home.

Raul turned to his counselor as the only person with whom he could talk about his anger and hurt at his mother's treatment of him. He admitted that if he was strong enough to go out and buy drugs. This is when he very much wanted to resume using cocaine. At the same time, he confided to his counselor that he was afraid that if he did resume taking drugs that would be the reason his mother would use for throwing him out of her apartment. He felt increasingly trapped and depressed.

Raul looked forward to coming to the clinic as the only place where he felt treated like a person. He used his counseling sessions to complain about his situation at home and discuss his feeling rejected and depressed. He resumed using cocaine and began to drink alcoholically. He became so sick that he was afraid to go to sleep, fearing that he would never again wake up. He became incoherent as a result of AIDS dementia and was readmitted to the hospital where he soon died.

Raul's mother was so angry at him and so ashamed that her son died from AIDS and had been a drug addict that initially she refused to make any of the plans for his funeral. Only after his counselor talked to her did she allow him to make arrangements under the guise of what would her friends and neighbors think when they learned that her son had died and there had not been a wake or mass.

In contrast to Raul, Ben already knew that he had been exposed to HIV when he applied to our program. He had spent two years in a therapeutic community recovering from his heroin addiction and was working as a counselor in a drug detoxification unit. It wasn't learning that he was seropositive that resulted in his relapsing into heroin use, but his fiance's breaking up with him as a result of his testing positive to HIV.

Ben's impending marriage and desire to father a child prompted him to take the HIV test. He knew that he was at risk for having been exposed to HIV but felt optimistic since he had not used drugs in over two years and was feeling fine. As a direct result of his having tested positive, his fiance moved out and ended their relationship. This hurt him so badly that he immediately resumed using heroin intravenously.

Ben's drug use began to affect his work performance, and he realized that he needed professional help. Having experienced recovery in a drug free modality, he was in a quandary about how to proceed. Unable to control his desire to use heroin to numb his pain, he finally decided to begin methadone maintenance. He applied and was accepted into our program.

During his initial counseling session at the program, Ben explained to his counselor how invested he had been in denying what his resumption of heroin meant. He also shared that he didn't know which frightened him more, heroin addiction or the possibility of developing AIDS. The counselor erroneously assumed that this level of honesty and insight meant that Ben had an excellent prognosis for stopping use of illicit drugs.

Ben's behavior after he resumed using heroin had been so erratic at his job that rumors began to circulate there that he was taking drugs. In addition to the stress of not feeling like he could be honest at his job about having begun methadone, Ben was feeling a high degree of stress from working each day with numerous chemically dependent clients who were either HIV positive or who had AIDS.

Ben's counselor was able to empathize with Ben's feelings about being HIV seropositive and working with chemically dependant clients who were struggling with these identical issues. The counselor shared his own status as a former i.v. drug user with Ben, as well as his own fears that perhaps he too was infected with HIV. These disclosures enabled Ben to open up and continue to make constructive use of the counseling sessions.

After entering our program Ben continued to have problems at work. He was chronically late as he had to pick up his methadone every day during clinic hours which made it impossible for him to arrive at work by the time he was supposed to be there. He refused to tell his supervisors why he had begun to be late. In addition, his job increasingly involved working with clients who had HIV illness. Eventually he just allowed himself to be fired from this job.

When exploring his having been fired from the job, the counselor realized two things. First, Ben had not been fully reporting to him how stressed he was by the situation at the job; second, the counselor had assumed that the little that Ben had shared with him had resulted in his exploring intrapsychically these same issues resulting in meaningful insight into the current stressors. The counselor's overidentification with Ben had caused him to incorrectly assess Ben as having more ego strength than in fact he possessed. The counselor realized that he should have been much more concrete and should have taken a problem solving approach, a method of working he attempted to employ from this point on.

Ben's being fired began a period of extremely impulsive and self-destructive behaviors. He charged a first class vacation for himself and his brother, assuming he would not live long enough to have to pay for it. He stopped paying rent, was evicted from his apartment, and destroyed his car in an accident. He refused to discuss whether the cause of this accident was related to his being high. During counseling sessions, Ben would use his anger and fatalism about getting AIDS and dying as a rationalization for the way he was behaving.

Recognizing how out of control Ben was, the counselor continued to have Ben come to the program six days a week for his methadone. This resulted in Ben's becoming very angry at his counselor. He'd tell his counselor that the only reasons he complied with the six day a week pick up schedule was that he didn't want to suffer from withdrawal from methadone and couldn't afford to buy street methadone. The counselor supported Ben's telling him all of these feelings both in individual and group counseling.

Ben moved in with his sister but moved out after two weeks because they had terrible arguments. He then moved in with his mother, but this arrangement didn't last long either. His mother asked him not to tell the man she lived with about his being exposed to HIV or about being on methadone. When Ben was ill, his mother would lie about his condition and say that he had cancer. She tried to be supportive and caring to Ben, but she was afraid that if the man she lived with found out that Ben had HIV, he would move out. This created tension between Ben and his mother which became an additional source of stress. Ben would share all of this with his counselor, making effective use of their sessions.

Ben would have preferred to move out but could not afford to do so until he found a furnished room within walking distance of his mother's house. This way he was able to visit often, have meals with her regularly, and see her for support when he was feeling anxious. She would often cook and send him home with extra food.

The winter of 1989 was very cold, and the rooming house was damp and often not well heated. Ben began to be constantly ill with severe colds or flu-like conditions as well as severe thrush which spread to his lips and made eating difficult and painful. To further complicate the situation, Ben would often not take the prescribed medication for these conditions. He claimed not to be able to afford many medications since he was now without health insurance.

But one thing that Ben decided he was able to afford was cocaine. By this time, Ben's income came from public assistance and he had medicaid which would pay for his prescribed medication. Yet he still did not follow the advice of his physicians. He was regularly being confronted by the counseling staff both about his use of cocaine and noncompliance with medical advice. Each time he was confronted by his counselor, he would change his behaviors just enough to not be discharged from the program.

Around the program, Ben was not secretive about having AIDS. Even before his condition progressed into full blown AIDS, he would often talk with other clients and staff about being exposed to HIV and the fact that his fiance left him because of this. Ben's sharing of this information resulted in his getting a lot of attention and sympathy from the other clients. When discussing either his health status or abandonment by his ex-fiance during counseling, Ben was never able to move past using this information in attempts to either elicit sympathy or manipulate staff to not be so hard on him.

Ben would only keep one out of every three or four scheduled medical appointments. He continued to refuse to take prescribed medication, saying that it could not cure him, made him feel worse and would only prolong his suffering. He began to lose weight since the thrush had spread to his esophagus and stomach, making eating very painful. The only food he could tolerate was cans of Nutriment. He refused to go to the gastro-intestinal clinic for an evaluation.

He became increasingly isolated, spending most of his time alone in his damp and poorly heated room. Ben complied with the barest minimum of the program policies so that he could continue to receive his methadone. One day he arrived at the clinic looking worse than usual, and the staff decided that he appeared too ill not to be sent to the emergency room. Ben was not given any methadone and told that after he was evaluated by medical personnel he could return for his methadone, or in the eventuality that he was admitted to the hospital, arrangements would be made for him to get it in the hospital. Though he was furious with the staff of our program, he had no alternative but to go to the emergency room. He died from pneumonia in the emergency room several hours later.

Every day people like Bea, Ben, and Raul are seen in methadone programs around the country. As difficult as their lives were, being on methadone and having access to counseling and medical care certainly made their lives better and easier than they would have been if they had never become clients of our program. Yet they are the lucky ones in so far as they were able to find a program that was able to help them. Thousands of people who want methadone or another form of treatment for their drug addiction are unable to receive help due to a shortage of treatment facilities.

When the difficult task of working with an addicted individual who is struggling with recovery is further complicated by HIV disease, treatment personnel in methadone clinics are challenged to the very limits of their expertise. The major goal of methadone maintenance is for the client to stop using illicit drugs, develop a productive life, and become a valued member of society. HIV is an additional assault to these clients' self-esteem and is often a new reason to resume taking nonprescribed drugs.

Bea, Raul, and Ben all had strong enough relationships with the program so that they continued to make use of the program's services when they didn't have the physical or psychic strength to go any place else. Despite various "acting out" behaviors, they and hundreds of other clients struggling with recovery from addiction, as well as from AIDS, were not rejected by the staff and were treated like human beings with a great many urgent needs. The methadone program became the point around which they organized their lives during their final days.

Since many of the staff of our program are individuals who themselves have a past history of drug addiction and are now in recovery and who may also be at risk for HIV infection, they understand and can empathize with the dilemmas and fears of our clients. Sometimes the program is the only place where our clients do not experience rejection and can bridge the isolation they so often feel.

Obviously the staff did not condone Raul's, Ben's, or Bea's use of cocaine or alcohol. When clients relapse into active substance abuse, their lives and the treatment obviously become more complicated. Drug-taking behavior on the part of the clients creates a lot of negative feelings towards them from some of the staff. Yet after carefully evaluating each case, the staff decided that discharging clients like Raul, Ben, and Bea from the program for using nonprescribed drugs would have probably resulted in shortening their lives. These clients would have been even more unlikely to avail themselves of medical interventions for their HIV conditions, and without methadone, their drug usage would certainly have escalated, increasing their exposure to various ailments that would have hastened their deaths. In addition, while in the program, these clients were exposed to safer needle use and safer sex information that may also have contributed to their not spreading HIV to other people. To this day the staff questions whether these are treatment failures or successes.

The additional stress that living with HIV illness places on an individual who is on methadone is frequently used as a rationalization for relapse into the use of nonprescribed substances. Obviously many clients with HIV on methadone become more depressed or anxious as their health deteriorates. For the most part, these are not people who have a history of tolerating intrapsychic distress. Their primary way of coping has been to take drugs.

Many of these clients have had the experience of physicians refusing to prescribe psychotropic medication once they learned that the client had a past history of addiction. This is often true even when the client is in great physical pain or obviously very depressed. Even upon learning that a client has been stable on methadone for a number of years with no evidence of illicit drug use, some physicians are reluctant to prescribe pain or mood altering medication. Thus many clients would rather not subject themselves to the possible humiliation of being refused needed medication and begin to self-medicate themselves with drugs they purchase on the streets.

For the three clients described above, relapse into drug use was a not unexpected coping strategy in response to HIV. As treatments for the opportunistic infections of AIDS improves and people with AIDS are living longer, staff is able to try and offer hope to clients with HIV. Hope is an essential component for clients to remain drug free. Even though none of the staff agreed with these clients' decisions to resume drug use, the staff understood the decisions and still maintained a caring relationship with each of these clients.

Most urban methadone programs have become experienced at working with clients whose lives are impacted by HIV. These programs provide an alternative to the rejection many clients experience from their families and friends. The programs provide one safe place for these very difficult and needy clients to discuss their fears and concerns. The challenges these clients present to staff are enormous. Yet by not rejecting these clients, we make a significant difference in their lives.

Chemical Dependency and Relapse in Gay Men with HIV Infection: Issues and Treatment

Darrell Greene, MA
Barbara Faltz, RN

There are two epidemics in the gay community—HIV infection and chemical dependency. Rates of chemical dependency are reported to be as much as three times higher for gay men (Pohl, 1988). Further, approximately one-third of all gay men are reported to be chemically dependent (Lohrenz, Connely, Coyne and Spare, 1978; Morales and Graves, 1984), and gay men are 14 to 28 times more likely to be diagnosed with AIDS relative to the general population (Fray, Turner, Klassen and Gagnon, 1989). Due to the proportion of gay men likely to be infected with HIV and the percentages of gay men demonstrating chemical dependency, it is evident that gay men with dual conditions of chemical dependency and HIV infection comprise a sizable population requiring counseling services and targeted intervention strategies.

These services are essential to gay men with HIV infection who are chemically dependent because of the life-threatening consequences of continued use. Three primary reasons may be identified which mandate counseling services: (1) For gay men with HIV infection whose chemical dependency remains untreated or who are in recovery and relapse, substance use may significantly exacerbate an already compromised immune system (MacGregor, 1987). (2) Reinfection or infection of others may occur as a function of disinhibition through substance use and noncompliance with risk reduction behaviors (Stall, 1988). (3) Progressive deterioration of the quality of life may occur for many men with HIV infection as for others diagnosed as chemically dependent. The gay man with

HIV infection and chemical dependency may lose his life from suicide, violence, automobile accidents, or medical complications long before experiencing any terminal symptomatic expression associated with AIDS.

While recent articles discuss the dual condition of chemical dependency and HIV infection (Faltz and Madover, 1987) and assessment procedures for gay men with chemical dependency (Faltz, 1988), little is available to the practitioner about comprehensive treatment approaches for gay men in recovery with HIV infection. This paper will discuss relapse prevention with providers involved in the treatment of chemical dependency in gay men with HIV seropositive status. Intervention strategies and a case illustration are presented to assist the counselor in providing services specific to the unique needs of gay men with HIV who are chemically dependent.

RELAPSE AND GAY MEN

The exploration of potential high risk events or stressors is essential to assisting clients in interrupting relapse conditions. For gay men, stressful events specific to the gay experience may promote relapse and require identification to provide effective relapse prevention counseling. Concerns of gay men, regardless of HIV status, potentially promoting relapse behavior are as follows:

1. *HIV associated distress*: The issues about HIV in gay men in general include fears of infection, coping with friends or lovers with HIV infection, losses due to AIDS, and sexual risk reduction compliance. All these issues may promote relapse in gay men given the distress of coping with the realities of present day gay experience.
2. *Internalized homophobia*: Simply as a function of being raised in the dominant culture, all gay men have at least some internalized negativity about their sexual identities. The awareness of internalized homophobia may escalate during abstinence from drugs and/or alcohol, and distress associated with a low self-image may promote relapse. Some gay men report feelings of alienation at general AA or NA meetings due to a perceived lack of support for differences in self-identity. How-

ever, gay men who have internalized negative self-images may also find it difficult to trust others of the same sexual orientation when this identity has been, in part, internally rejected.

3. *External homophobia*: Gay men suffer stigma and discrimination from others when their sexual identity is known or suspected. Family, friends, and co-workers may react with overt or subtle rejection of gays. Further, direct or indirect discrimination by unknown others in terms of politics or "fag-bashing" may induce feelings of anger and anguish in general. These feelings may be experienced as difficult to cope with by the gay man in recovery and possibly promote relapse into substance use. Finally, gay men who divide themselves by "passing" as heterosexual in the dominant culture may experience tremendous stress, both by living inauthentically and fearing discovery. Clearly, the "environmental hostility" of the present society may be associated with relapse.

4. *Socialization*: Contact with other gay men often occurs in gay bars, and in many parts of the country, this is the only place for gays to freely meet other gays. Given this environment, however, "triggers" promoting relapse for gay men in recovery are highly apparent. Peers who are not in recovery may unwittingly encourage the chemically dependent gay man to use again. As socialization with other gay men may be restricted in some communities, the gay man in recovery may be highly isolated. Without the development of alternative social involvements, relapse may be likely for gay men in recovery.

5. *Disrupted life areas*: Prior to engaging in treatment, gay men's chemical dependency may have significantly disrupted life areas of social and intimate relationships, vocational functioning, finance, and physical health. The lack of restitution in these areas tend to be predictive of relapse in gay men who feel overwhelmed by their circumstances and lack support systems to assist in the progressive management of the consequences of prerecovery behavior.

6. *Function of substance use*: Gay men may use substances for a number of self-defined purposes. Control over mood states, thought processes, or behavior may be perceived as available

through substance use. For example, gay men who have difficulty socializing with peers may employ chemicals to increase their assertiveness or reduce inhibitions. Further, substance use may be employed to allow for behaviors about which some gay men may feel uncomfortable or unwilling to assume responsibility. This may be particularly true for gay men with difficulty accepting same-sex sexual contact. Chemical use in the general community may also be used as a symbol of celebration and to distinguish situations from everyday events. Similarly, gay men may employ substances to disassociate from the pressures of the dualities of their lives or to make a statement of transition from generally-presented to gay-presented identities. Finally, substance use may be employed as a statement of differentiation from the majority or "straight" culture and be perceived as an expression of openness to experience "masculine-identity," heightened sensuality, or disregard for societal rules. Without the development of skills perceived as solely available through substance use and the reintegration of gay identity in abstinence, relapse is likely for gay men.

RELAPSE AND GAY MEN
WITH HIV INFECTION

In addition to high risk events or stressors promoting relapse for gay men generally, the practitioner must be aware of triggers for relapse specific to gay men with HIV infection. These triggers for relapse include issues of hopelessness, bargaining, medical care, self-blame, and stigmatization.

Hopelessness: Gay men in recovery who become aware of their seropositive status may experience acute reactions of anxiety or depression. Regardless of appropriate pretest counseling, the gay man in recovery may interpret his test result as a "death sentence" (Levine, 1989). For many, HIV seropositive status notification may stimulate a questioning of the value and meaning of abstention from alcohol and/or drugs. The gay man with HIV infection may ask himself "why bother" to initiate or maintain recovery now that he perceives his "life has been taken" from him. Through "euphoric recall" he may also imagine using substances as a mechanism to ease emotional distress or returning to the "pleasures" of substance use while he is able to do so. These thoughts may reoccur and intensify as the gay man with HIV infection experiences the ongoing traumas associated with HIV infection and struggles with what he believes himself capable of tolerating.

A "why bother" mentality may also be expressed by significant others or professional providers to chemically dependent gay men with HIV infection (Faltz and Madover, 1988). Chemical dependency may be overlooked or facilitated by prescription medications or other forms of enabling in an attempt to "assist" the client with enduring his illness. Clearly, this response by medical or social systems may reinforce the client's hopelessness through messages of permission for self-destructiveness by continued substance abuse.

Bargaining: In contrast to feelings of hopelessness, some gay men may react to HIV seropositive status as an opportunity to improve the quality of their lives and fortify their determination to abstain or initiate treatment. This response may reflect an unconscious bargaining with their health status, with the hope that nonuse will prevent initial or further symptomatic expression. However, as disease manifestations occur, or other HIV-related traumatization are experienced, risk of relapse becomes acute. The gay man with HIV infection may return to substance abuse as he feels unable to control the circumstances of his life, and a resumption of substance use becomes a metaphor for feelings of powerlessness.

Medical care: The taking of medications for HIV, even those as innocuous as antiviral drugs, has been described by many gay men with chemical dependency histories as producing recollections of past drug taking and stimulating thoughts of resuming use. Prescription medications for pain or stimulants to improve concentration may "set up" clients with histories of chemical dependency for excessive self-medicating and relapse. Average doses of opiates may not be successful in relieving pain in gay men with a history of substance abuse because of high tolerance levels. This may again encourage clients to return to chemical abuse in an attempt at self-management of physical distress.

Self-blame: Self-negativity may intensify for gay men with HIV infection in recovery as the client blames himself for his health status. Unless imagined culpability for HIV infection and associated guilt is addressed, the potential for relapse in this population is significantly increased.

Stigmatization: While external homophobia may be cushioned through the support of one's peers, the multiple stigmatization of those with chemical dependency and HIV infection may be experienced within the gay community. As social support may become increasingly restricted for the gay man with HIV infection and chemical dependency, isolation may be profound. Even in areas where AA meetings are organized within the gay community, the gay man in recovery with HIV infection may be highly reluctant to "come out" with his health status.

RELAPSE PREVENTION IN GAY MEN WITH HIV INFECTION

A number of intervention strategies may be employed to assist gay men with HIV infection to sustain their recovery and interrupt relapse potential. It is not unusual for gay men who are in recovery to express feeling hopeless when they learn that they are infected with HIV or have been diagnosed with an AIDS related opportunistic infection. Not infrequently these feelings become rationalizations for a desire to resume using alcohol or drugs. Counselors working with gay men who are expressing these kinds of feelings need to empathize with them and explain to the clients that thoughts of picking up drugs or alcohol are normal during the kind of stressful situation they are currently going through. Yet this a time that the counselor must also be very directive in helping the client use the tools he has learned within twelve-step programs and therapy so that instead of acting out on these feelings he can tolerate the feelings without medicating himself.

It is only natural that those with a chemical dependency history would define an "escape clause" should the physical and emotional pain of HIV disease exceed the client's level of tolerance. Talking about "getting high again" is equivalent to other clients with HIV infection imagining a semblance of control over their circumstances through suicidal ideation. Further, just as with a suicidal assessment, the counselor would ascertain the concreteness of a "relapse plan." Questions of how the client would use, present access to substances, and when he might lapse will provide the counselor with important information as to the imminence of relapse potential and will direct intervention strategies accordingly.

For the majority of gay men imagining a return to use, the counselor may assist the client in reframing this option as an expression of affective distress and encourage client verbalizations of underlying fear, pain, frustration, or anguish. Additionally, the client may be helped by attending to the fact that thoughts are not necessarily tied to action. Finally, the communication of affect and other methods of coping may be explored as alternatives to substance use in dealing with distress throughout the therapeutic process.

When clients' thoughts of relapse are associated with a direct plan of action, the counselor may offer guidance to the client by developing an alternative plan and confronting the client with the potential consequences of returning to substance use. Involvement in AA or NA and contact with sponsors may be structured, as well as other activities interrupting relapse potential.

Bargaining strategies utilized as a psychological "safeguard" against symptomatic expression may motivate clients to initiate treatment or maintain recovery and in early treatment should not be interrupted. However, discussion of potential triggers to relapse must invariably include identification of the potential for symptoms of HIV related illnesses to occur and other emotionally distressing events to assist clients in preparing for all traumatic possibilities. For many, this will elicit responses of anxiety, dysphoria, and hopelessness, and interventions of normalization or structured planning may be introduced.

As medical regimes may be a strong trigger for relapse, contracting of dose levels, and information sharing between physician, client, and counselor is strongly recommended. Further, relapse potential may be interrupted when the client is assured of adequate medical intervention by the treatment team to relieve painful symptomatic expressions.

Self-blame for HIV infection is often associated with a client's chemical dependency and creates feelings of low self-worth and intense shame or guilt. These feelings may dramatically interfere with a client's ability to adjust to his condition and sustain recovery. Client self-blame for HIV infection may be redirected by attending to their lack of intentionality, in addition to identifying the effects of the disease of chemical dependency on their lives. As blame is shifted from the self to the disease of chemical dependency, client motivation to maintain treatment may be heightened.

Finally, stigmatization for HIV seropositive status and chemical dependency may exist within both the dominant culture and the gay community. Further, AIDS anxiety and homophobia within the recovery community may discourage self-disclosure for the gay man with HIV infection attending AA or NA meetings and may even prevent him from informing his sponsor about his health status. Clearly, as the gay man with HIV infection and chemical dependency disassociates from his program of recovery, relapse into substance use can usually be predicted. For many, the process of sharing HIV status reflects a reexperiencing of "coming out" about gay identities and chemical dependency. It is imperative that the counselor assist in the development of a support network for gay clients with HIV infection and chemical dependency.

In addition to issues about revealing health status, some gay men with HIV infection in recovery feel "disloyal" to or unwelcomed by their recovery program when taking necessary and prescribed medication for psychological or physical distress. The counselor may facilitate support by encouraging clients to participate in gay recovery meetings designed for those who are HIV infected, such as Positives Anonymous or Triple A (AA and AIDS) meetings. If this form of recovery meeting is unavailable, counselor understanding and support and the promotion of sponsor awareness through therapeutic involvement with the client becomes essential to sustained involvement in treatment and abstention for gay clients engaged in recovery.

In addition to assessing and treating specific manifestations of hopelessness, bargaining, medical care, self-blame, and stigmatization associated with gay men with HIV infection in recovery, general issues confronting all gay men in chemical dependency treatment must be addressed in order to interrupt relapse potential. These general issues include HIV associated distress, internalized homophobia, external homophobia, socialization, disrupted life areas, and function of substance use. While complex, counselor attention to these factors may assist gay male clients with HIV infection to sustain their recovery. Through an assessment of these issues, the client and practitioner may define strategies to promote client well-being. The following case illustration is presented to provide the counselor with an example of assessment procedures and the development of intervention strategies specific to gay men with HIV infection in recovery.

CASE ILLUSTRATION: JOHN A.

John A. is a twenty-eight year-old gay white poly-chemical abuser with HIV seropositivity, who has been actively involved in AA for one year. Through this period he has been able to maintain his abstinence. John had been unemployed until six months ago, living on unemployment compensation, as he had been fired from his job as a salesman. Presently, he is working as a waiter in a local restaurant and finds satisfaction in the job but anticipates a return to sales once he feels more "stable."

John initiated his chemical dependency recovery a few weeks after losing his job. He reports choosing to get tested after a close friend and former sex partner died from AIDS. While others in his recovery group are HIV seropositive, John has been unable to reveal his health status to them or to his sponsor, although his sponsor is aware of his gay identity. He reports fearing that he would "be seen differently" by them if they were to know his status and is concerned that his "confidentiality would be compromised" if "word was out" about him.

The only people who are aware of John's seropositivity are his doctor and counselor. John reports monitoring his blood levels every few months. His most recent medical assessment revealed a decline in his helper T cells, and his doctor has encouraged John to begin AZT treatment. This has been agonizing for John, and he reports feeling a sense of frustration that he could become symptomatic regardless of having become sober. He states that he knew he could "get sick" anyway but hoped that not using would "protect" him for "at least a few years." His recent medical report has stimulated thoughts of using again, as well as memories of his friend that died of AIDS related infections. These thoughts had motivated John to involve himself in counseling.

John reports using alcohol and other drugs historically to "relax" due to severe anxiety when he was 18 years old and coming out in gay bars. Through substance use John was able to establish relationships with others that he described as focused upon "getting high rather than talking." Further, he disclosed being uncomfortable with "having sex" and would "get loaded" when wanting to be sexual. These encounters were associated with a great deal of self-recrimination, and John identified feeling "miserable" afterwards and "even more alone." Since engaging in recovery, John has been sexually abstinent, both as a function of an inability to "connect" with others and fears about reinfection or infecting others with HIV. Additionally, John reports a great deal of guilt about his HIV status, as he "occasionally practiced unsafe sex" when intoxicated.

In assessing John's relapse potential, he reports "sometimes wanting to get high again," and that these thoughts are particularly intense when thinking about "what might happen" to him physically, remembering the loss of his friend, or when feeling lonely. While John has been able to cope with these thoughts by "going to a meeting" or "calling his sponsor," he is aware of an increased need "to talk with somebody about being HIV positive."

When the counselor explored John's feelings about past experiences being sexual with other men he reported sex was "easy" for him when using substances, but that now that he is clean and sober, he feels "very uncomfortable" with sex. He believes he could practice safer sex if he had the opportunity, but sometimes feels a sense of "self-disgust" when imagining sexual activity in which he has participated in the past. John feels particularly ambivalent about anal sex and defines this discomfort as, in part, separate from his fears about HIV infection. While consciously believing that any form of sexual expression as being "okay," he reports feeling self-critical of his own desires.

The counselor and client identified the need to assist John in developing social supports with other gay men who are in recovery, or who will encourage his recovery, with whom he can also discuss his HIV status and concerns. To promote this goal, the counselor and client contracted to: practice informing his sponsor and others of his health status; engage his sponsor in treatment; promote social skill development; increase self-acceptance; and develop techniques to reduce anxiety in general. In addition to these goals, the counselor emphasized the importance of John's recovery program as a primary condition for maintaining his sobriety. Finally the counselor and John agreed to explore issues of sexual expression and loss once John has been able to achieve initial counseling goals.

CONCLUSIONS

Through the analysis of presenting concerns and situational stressors, the counselor and client were able to identify areas requiring immediate attention and develop a plan for future treatment. This allowed the practitioner and client an opportunity to interrupt the potential for relapse by assisting the client in developing alternative means of coping with distress.

While techniques of treatment for relapse prevention, in terms of coping skill acquisition or enhancement and identification of situations associated with "risk" are similar for gay men, regardless of HIV status, the unique conditions of distress that may lead to relapse in gay men who are HIV positive must be appreciated by the counselor in order to provide effective treatment for this population. Without a willingness by the counselor to explore in detail and without judgment, the issues specific to gay men in recovery with HIV infection, the likelihood of client success in maintaining recovery may be significantly reduced. Treatment programs and individual providers must do more than not assume all men in recovery are heterosexual or HIV negative; they must offer a safe and supportive atmosphere for all clients to explore their unique concerns about maintaining abstinence.

REFERENCES

Faltz, B. (1988). "Substance abuse and the lesbian and gay community: assessment and intervention." In M. Shernoff and W. Scott (Eds.) *The Sourcebook on Lesbian/Gay Health Care*, Washington, D.C.: National Lesbian/Gay Health Foundation, 151-161.

Faltz, B. and Madover, S. (1987). "Treatment of substance abuse in patients with HIV infection." *Advances in Alcohol and Substance Abuse*, 7(2), 143-157.

Fray, R.E., Turner, C.F., Klassen, A.D., and Gaynon, J.H. (1989). "Prevalence and patterns of same-sex contact among men." *Science*, 243(4889), 338-348.

Levine, C. (1989). "AIDS and drug use: breaking the link." *AIDS Education and Prevention*, 1(3), 231-246.

Lohrenz, L.F., Connley, J.C., Coyne, L. and Spare, K.E. (1978). "Alcohol problems in several midwestern homosexual communities." *Journal of Studies on Alcohol*, 39(11), 1959-1963.

MacGregor, R.R. (1987). "Alcohol and drugs as co-factors for AIDS." In L. Siegel (Ed.) *AIDS and Substance Abuse*. New York: Harrington Park Press, 47-72.

Morales, E.S. and Graves, M.A. (1983). *Substance Abuse: Patterns and Barriers to Treatment for Gay Men and Lesbians in San Francisco*. San Francisco: Department of PUblic Health Community Substance Abuse Services, 16-25.

Stall, R. (1988). "The prevention of HIV infection associated with drug and alcohol use during sexual activity." In L. Siegel (Ed.) *AIDS and Substance Use*, New York: Harrington Park Press, 73-80.

Care of HIV Infected Native American Substance Abusers

Ronald M. Rowell, MPH
Hannah Kusterer, MS, MFCC

The Friendship House Association of American Indians is a 20 bed 6 month (90 days residential, 90 days aftercare) drug and alcohol treatment program in the Mission District of San Francisco. It receives its primary funding from the Indian Health Service and the City of San Francisco. Ninety-percent of its clients are Native American. It serves as a regional treatment program for not only the San Francisco Bay Area, but for rural Northern California and Northern Nevada also. In 1990, it received recognition from the Indian Health Service as a model program for the nation.

Although not often thought of as cities with significant Indian populations, San Francisco and Oakland were sites for Indian relocation during the 1950s, when the Federal Government's policy moved Indian people from rural/reservation areas to cities where they hoped Indians would be assimilated. Because of its location, the program often serves gay/bisexual Indians who have come to San Francisco to live freely, the same as gay/bisexual people of other ethnicities have done. Other Indian people come to the area in hope of finding work, because family members or friends live here, or for some, because their drug of choice is more accessible. The gender make-up of the client population in the program varies, but generally the residents are about 60% men and 40% women.

The clinical staff of Friendship House have been trained as HIV/AIDS educators and organizers through the National Native American AIDS Prevention Program in Oakland. HIV/AIDS prevention education is integrated into the recovery program, and each client is required to participate. Clinical staff also act as supplemental pre- and post-HIV antibody test counselors for clients who are considering or who choose to get tested and wish more in depth counseling than is available at alternative test sites. Staff from the American Indian AIDS Institute in San Francisco are occasionally called upon for assistance with client education.

Friendship House treats both drug and alcohol abusers. The clientele can be divided into three primary groups: those whose drug of choice is only alcohol; those who use only drugs intravenously; and those who use alcohol and drugs combined. Proportionally, those who are only alcoholic make up on average 20% of the residents at any given time. Those who are IVDUs make up 45%. Those who are poly-substance abusers another 35%. Of the latter, a third have used drugs intravenously at some point in their lives, not just once but on a sustained basis.

Patterns which we believe are specifically Native American have emerged from our work with each of these groups. There are people who do not fit these categories, but we have chosen these because we believe they are indicative of those in the program most at-risk of HIV infection. Although drug abuse is also a problem on reservations, the majority of our clients who come from reservations abuse alcohol only. (Only one out of four Native Americans resides on a reservation.) They have had their first drink as children; for example, drinking beer left over from a parent's party the night before. Their families tend to be alcoholic, but ties with the family are close, if dysfunctional. Heavy drinking is considered a normal part of life, and recovery is difficult when there is nothing to go home to which isn't partying. Someone in the person's family has most likely died from a vehicular accident or fight as a result of being under the influence. These individuals tend to come into treatment as a result of a court-ordered referral or because they are threatened with loss of their children. They also tend to be closer to their tribal traditions and more likely to speak their tribal language. Neither males nor females predominate in this category.

Gay/bisexual male clients seen at Friendship House most often fit into the "only alcoholic" category. At Friendship House they are more likely to have been living on the street as indigents. They have often been turning tricks in order to find a warm bed to sleep in.

Many times the men come into the program off the street via 72-hour detox. They will often have had serial relationships — perhaps more properly termed serial sexual encounters since they are commercial in nature.

Gay/bisexual men and lesbians often have a hard time with other clients in the program. There is often a negative verbal reaction in groups to the mention of gay and lesbian Indians or HIV/AIDS. While this is true when these topics are brought up as abstract ideas, the attitude often changes once a client has come out to the group and the issue becomes personalized. In our experience, those often the most vehement in their condemnations of gays and lesbians have been sexually abused as children, particularly men sexually abused by other men. They have made an association in their mind between molestation and homosexuality, and their anger prevents them from understanding the very real distinction between homosexual orientation and sexual abuse. Most of the gay clients are "out" in their lives within the gay community of San Francisco, but not back home. Sexual orientation issues come up in individual counseling sessions. Only about half the gay/lesbian clients choose to come out in group sessions among other Indians, almost always reluctantly.

Most lesbian clients seen at Friendship House have fit into the IVDU category, although some are alcoholic as well. They are more likely to have lived on the street than female alcoholic or poly-drug clients and more likely to have turned tricks with heterosexual men to survive.

The majority of IV drug users seen at Friendship House use heroin as the drug of choice and nothing else. These clients often have sexual abuse and other trauma as a precipitating factor in their move to inject. They have usually already used marijuana and alcohol prior to injecting. The average age of beginning IV drug use is 12 or 13 years old, often immediately after a rape or molestation episode. They have generally experienced more encounters with the law and have served time in jail for felony convictions. They are frequently separated from their families of origin and from children. "Estranged" is the word we would use to summarize their relationships in general. Whether this is due to the fact that it may be easier to support their habit in the big city or whether their families couldn't stand living with their habit, we don't know. They are much more transient than the other clients, often having lived in several states and cities. They are also more apt to have lived on the street and to have turned tricks to support their habit.

Poly-substance abusers are much more difficult to typify. Among these, we also see trauma and encounters with law enforcement, but also people who are able to live relatively functional lives. There is a fairly wide spectrum of individuals in this classification in our program. This is the category into which most of the clients we see who use crack appear to fit.

Prostitution among our clients tends to be among the gay male alcoholics, lesbian IV drug users, and heterosexual women IVDUs or crack users. The prostitution of which we are speaking cannot be thought of as professional but as a direct result of an individual's habit. Although we suspect that a portion of our heterosexual male clients may also have engaged in male-male prostitution for drugs or money, none of these clients has ever admitted to doing so in either individual or group therapy in our memory.

In general, our Indian IVDU clients appear to have greater knowledge of how HIV is transmitted and often are already either not sharing their kits or are cleaning them with bleach and water. Gay male clients, even though generally well-versed in HIV transmission, appear to be having much more difficulty with changing sexual practices which place them at risk. These alcoholic gay Indian men seem to have no history of functional relationships. When they are involved, often they feel emotionally powerless and are often victimized. They are simply unable or unwilling to consider their own needs.

The majority of our clients come into the program with little knowledge about AIDS and with many misconceptions about how HIV is transmitted. Fear of casual infection is the most common issue we deal with when clients first participate in discussions or education about AIDS. In order to overcome this misinformation, weekly HIV/AIDS education is integrated into the treatment plan. Clients often have difficulty trusting the HIV/AIDS information they are given in the program. This mistrust is attributable to the clients' own substance abuse and being reared in abusing families. It is especially a problem for those who have lived parts of their lives on the street. For Indian clients, the association of AIDS information and guidelines with the U.S. Government creates an even bigger barrier to trust. Many Indian clients feel that the U.S. Government has never been truthful in its relationship with the indigenous nations of North America, so why should it be trusted concerning AIDS information?

The following case studies provide a cross-section of American Indian clients infected with HIV treated for substance abuse at Friendship House. They also provide examples of many of the issues discussed above. The information in this article is aimed at programs which are not specifically targeted to Native American clients but which may have Native American clients in their caseload.

At Friendship House, most of our residents are at risk for exposure to HIV. Among our clientele are gay and lesbian men and women, IV drugs users, and partners of IVDUs. Nearly everyone who comes through the program has had multiple sexual partners during periods of heavy drug and alcohol use. Most of our clients have been sexually abused as children and have poor limit-setting skills, even when they know they are taking a risk. Often clients, both men and women, have prostituted themselves when they have had nowhere to stay or no money for drugs. In order to protect the confidentiality of our clients, some details have been changed. No individual's identity, therefore, can be assumed from these descriptions.

CASE STUDY ONE: JACK

Jack is a 30-year-old Crow man from Montana. He took his first drink when he was 6, finishing up beers left by partying adults. His whole family is alcoholic. He has two older sisters and a brother. His father was violent and died five years ago. He was raised by his sister and was molested by an uncle and a neighbor when he was eleven. He was a loner when he was younger and was beaten up and made fun of by the other kids. Eventually Jack left his home area and moved to the city. He has been moving around a lot since then and does not really feel that he can return home, although he would like to be able to. Jack is gay and feels that his family has rejected him because of being "different."

In the urban life, Jack's alcoholism has progressed rapidly. When necessary, he has sex with men to get a place to stay. He has spent a lot of time on the street and has been beaten so badly that he will do anything to keep a living arrangement intact. He has been in abusive alcoholic relationships and has an ulcer from stress, but no other evident medical problems. While he knows about AIDS, he really doesn't care if he lives or dies; in fact, he has attempted suicide twice. He has had periods of maintaining sobriety but has relapsed when he tries to visit home. Currently his only family contact is with his older sister. He was raised within his tribe's traditions, but he has a lot of conflict about how he has been treated and has a hard time accepting himself as a gay Indian. This client has had multiple sexual partners and also knows that some of his former lovers are sick with AIDS now. He worked in a bathhouse for a while and often had sex while in an alcoholic blackout.

As Jack progresses further in treatment, he is exposed to AIDS information while sober. Also, he is beginning to deal for the first time with some of his experiences of abuse as a child and is beginning to become emotionally self-aware. He is scared. He begins to talk with one of the counselors about taking the HIV antibody test. He has been unwilling to let the group know that he is gay, both from the fear of being treated as he was as a child and because others in the group have expressed hateful attitudes about gays. In addition, several people have expressed during the AIDS group their fear of having to live in the same house as someone with AIDS. Although the group is emphatically taught that there is no risk to them from casual contact, some doubt remains, and Jack expresses his conviction that he would be shunned if anyone even suspected he might be infected.

He is encouraged to deal with his feelings as openly as possible but is also supported in choosing if and when to do so. He insists that the counselor promise not to tell anyone, including other staff about his thinking about being tested. He sometimes threatens to leave the program if he thinks that he is making someone else uncomfortable. In his individual sessions, he discusses his fears about the test and possibly being HIV positive. He is told to take it one day at a time and not to upset himself about what might happen in the future. He is reminded as well that even a positive test is not an AIDS diagnosis and that if he stays sober and takes care of himself, he could have many quality years before becoming sick, if ever. He might even be well long enough for a cure to be found. He is also reminded that it does not matter if he knows his HIV status — what matters is changing his behavior. He should not consider testing if the knowledge would interfere with his sobriety.

After a few weeks of discussing these issues in private, Jack surprises his counselor with the news that he has been tested and will get the results in two weeks. He insists again that no one else be told about it and withdraws a bit from the group. He jokes a lot and doesn't have much to say about how he feels while waiting for his test results. He doesn't allow himself any support. On the day his test results are due, he insists he prefers to go by himself even though the counselor offers to accompany him and encourages him to accept the support. Jack does not come back.

CASE STUDY TWO: MARK

Mark is another typical client. He is a Klamath Indian from Oregon. He is 34 years old and has been a heroin addict for 15 years. He has used drugs and alcohol since he was 13 years old. He has tried to clean up a few times, or at least control his habit, but has used alcohol and pot constantly during these attempts. Mark's father, also an addict/alcoholic, was killed in a fight when Mark was four. His alcoholic mother was abusive and unable to take care of her three children. At the age of five, Mark was separated from his siblings and placed in a white fundamentalist Christian foster home, where he was brutally beaten.

Mark has a wife and two children, but he has not seen them for seven years, although he sends a little support now and then. His wife used to use drugs too but began to clean up when she became pregnant with their second child. He still thinks they will get back together when he decides to settle down. He met his current girlfriend in a recovery program. After two weeks, they left together, and within three months, they were both using. When a relationship becomes intimate, Mark gets angry and usually walks out before he gets violent, he says. He immediately gets into another relationship, and he is pretty clear about using women to take care of his needs. Although he is unaware of this, he uses sex to fix his feelings in much the same way he uses heroin.

Mark has been in prison twice, once for armed robbery and once for assault. He is streetwise, tough and angry, and doesn't care with whom he shoots up. He never uses any precautions during sex and leaves a woman if she starts making demands. At the beginning of the HIV/AIDS education group, he belligerently asks why he has to learn about this when he isn't gay. Later, he expresses a lot of anger toward gays. His anger is so intense that the staff speculates that Mark, who has a trim body and long hair, was raped in prison.

As Mark's treatment progresses, he begins to recognize his softer side and the hurt and pain beneath his anger. He has to be helped to slow down, to learn to contain these feelings without shutting down, as these are the feelings he uses drugs to avoid. His treatment turns a corner when he remembers spending time with his grandfather when he was very young and being taught about life with love and gentleness. For the first time, he begins exploring more of his heritage and seriously considers getting in touch with his family. He begins to attend a weekly sweat lodge. He is helped to contact his tribe and is making progress in dealing with his extensive legal problems. He starts thinking about writing to his children.

Mark is worried about his HIV status, now that he has been willing to acknowledge that he is not only at-risk, but that he has something to live for after all. He states that if he is HIV positive, he would definitely go out and use and probably just kill himself rather than go through all that suffering. However, if he's negative, he really wants to know and not have to think and worry about it. This client discusses his dilemma openly in the group and receives a lot of support from everyone. He is given the same information as Jack, and he decides that he can postpone testing until a later time when he may be better able to deal with the news. He does not want to risk his recovery.

However, he also still does not want to use a condom and doesn't know how to handle the knowledge that he could potentially be infecting his partner. Mark is angry about the choices he has to make, and as he always does when he is angry and feels cornered, he wants just to walk away.

CASE STUDY THREE: CHARLENE

Charlene is a 25 year-old Pomo woman from California, with one eight year old daughter who lives with her aunt. Charlene is an alcoholic and heroin addict and a lesbian. She never really knew her father, and her alcoholic mother always had a lot of different boyfriends over to the house. Charlene, the only daughter, was abused sexually by two of these "uncles," as well as by several other people. When she told her mother, her mother called her a slut and didn't believe her. She got most of her support from her aunt, who now has custody of Charlene's daughter. This aunt is a Christian and doesn't use drugs or alcohol and represents the only emotional safety this client has ever known.

Charlene has several issues to face. She is court-ordered to complete a program to regain custody of her daughter. She has court fines to pay and is on probation for three years. Two of her brothers are in jail, and one died of an overdose last year. She is really angry with her mother, and her aunt is not in very good health. She has no job skills and is confused about her feelings about her lover. When she was on her own, she was living in the city and was working the streets as a prostitute to maintain her habit. She is sick, tired, and run down. She did not take safety precautions during sex with customers and has been treated for STDs twice. She does, however, use her own works and refuses to share with anyone. She remembers having shared on a few occasions though, and she is afraid she might have been infected with HIV as a result. She has quite a bit of information about AIDS and has even been tested, with negative results. She wants to be tested again and is clear that she would rather know than wonder.

This client talks openly during group about her feelings about getting tested and is able to support others who have not been tested but are considering it. She is unable to talk openly about being a lesbian. She is afraid that the women will reject her. On the other hand, several of the men are giving her attention and letting her know they are attracted to her, and this frightens her very much, as she feels tremendous pressure from this attention.

The HIV antibody test is not a central issue for this client. She is tested, and although a bit anxious, is found to be negative. An issue that could continue to put her at risk, however, is an inability to set firm limits with other people. If someone wants something from her, she doesn't know how to refuse. This problem, stemming from her childhood abuse, is at the core of her addiction. Even slight pressure from others causes her to feel invaded and overwhelmed — and she only knows how to escape through drugs.

We worked with her extensively on developing other choices, and she made a lot of progress in the program. She was able to end the relationship she was in when her lover resumed using. She went to take care of her aunt and was doing well with her daughter. She joined her aunt's church and was finding that having a spiritual support system was very helpful. After one year, she relapsed when she found out that a relative had molested her daughter. However, after two months, she got into a program again and is still clean and sober today.

There are very many elements in common between American Indian people in treatment for substance abuse and people of other ethnic backgrounds. There are also many elements in common between HIV infected American Indian people and others. The following are some issues which we believe are specifically "Indian" which clients bring with them into the program.

POST-TRAUMATIC STRESS SYNDROME

The consequences of five hundred years of contact with and domination by peoples from Europe are still with us. Phil Tingley, past Chair of the American Indian Social Workers, has referred to these consequences as similar to the post-traumatic stress syndrome (PTSD) identified among men who have been in battle (Tingley, 1989). PTSD is the normal human reaction to severe trauma, shock, or pain. It can also affect those in close interpersonal relationships with such individuals and can have intergenerational consequences.

Perhaps the most severe trauma suffered by Native peoples was the demographic collapse of the Native American population due to epidemics of infectious disease. These diseases included small pox, typhoid, typhus, influenza, and syphilis among others. The population nadir occurred at the turn of the century when there were fewer than 300,000 Native people, from a 1492 population estimated at between 12 and 15 million. The fact that today there are an estimated 1.7 million is a tribute to the ability of Native people to survive.

One of the ways Native people survived was by taking care of their own no matter what occurred. This strategy was particularly effective at the time it arose in response to outside stress. Now, however, it has led to a dysfunctional enmeshment among some families.

In traditional Native societies boundaries were clear concerning what was acceptable and unacceptable individual behavior within the society. Many of these boundaries were blurred in response to the historical crisis faced by Indian people. What once was a survival mechanism is no longer functional. Where the system becomes dysfunctional is when alcohol and drugs enter the picture. The taking care of one's own no matter what enables individuals to continue their abuse. The result is codependency which does not help to heal or promote healthy behavior.

SPIRITUAL/CULTURAL FOUNDATION BUILDING

A sense of spiritual connection and awareness is extremely important in virtually all Native American cultures. The challenge is to help American Indian clients to reconnect with their culture, what we refer to as spiritual foundation building. For Indian clients spirituality does not necessarily mean going to church on Sundays. It means being connected to the family in healthy ways, to the land, to the clan, to the tribe way of life. American Indian traditional spirituality is woven into everything a person is or does. For clients at Friendship House, traditional Native American spirituality is often expressed through attendance at sweat lodge ceremonies. The Red Road approach to recovery as taught by Gene Thin Elk is an excellent example of how traditional spirituality can be used with

Native substance abusers and is incorporated into the Friendship House model of care. The Red Road approach involves using Native American symbols and metaphors to reinterpret the twelve-step program into a more culturally-specific model of recovery.

Culture and spirituality are tightly interwoven for Native American people. The film "The Honor of All," produced by the Alkali Lake Band of Shuswap in British Columbia illustrates better than anything else the importance of culture to recovery. The film is the story of how one reserve went from being virtually all alcoholic to 95% sober in the period of ten years. It is acted by the people who experienced it. A major tool and outcome of the recovery process was the reintegration of traditional rituals into the daily life of the community.

Ritual helps to set parameters and contain emotional responses within a limited arena. The sweat lodge, for example, allows emotional release in a safe environment, helping to enable an individual to master him/herself. In all tribal traditions, ritual and prayer have played a very important role in the healing process. Prayer is a recognition of our connection to a higher power, the life force of all things in the cosmos.

Any program working with HIV infected Native American substance abusers must be able to offer access to traditional Native spiritual resources. This can be done by networking with agencies which provide services specifically to Native Americans.

AIDS AMONG NATIVE AMERICANS

The absolute numbers of reported AIDS cases among Native Americans is relatively low in comparison with other ethnic groups. This may be due either to a later entrance of HIV into the population or to underreporting. A study by the Centers for Disease Control of reported Native American AIDS cases in Los Angeles and Seattle found on average that four out of five cases were misreported as Hispanic or White. Nevertheless, rates of sexually transmitted diseases remain twice as high for Native Americans as for the U.S. as a whole and preliminary reports from seroprevalence surveys among Native Americans shows rates of infection much higher than expected based upon the reported AIDS cases. Based on this information, we can expect to be faced with many more HIV infected clients in Native American substance abuse treatment programs in the years to come.

REFERENCE

Tingley, P. (1989). In E. Duran, (Ed.). "Post-Traumatic Stress Behavior: A Foundation for Suicide?" *Suicide Handbook: Prevention and Intervention With Native Americans*. San Francisco: Friendship House Association of American Indians, Inc., 51-58.

Counseling Incarcerated Individuals with HIV Disease and Chemical Dependency

Donald McVinney, CAC

This paper will address counseling incarcerated individuals with the dual diagnosis of chemical dependency and HIV disease. While the number of incarcerated individuals with HIV disease and a history of chemical dependency is unknown, it has been estimated that between 50% to 85% of all individuals who are incarcerated have a prior history of alcohol and other drug use (New York State Department of Health AIDS Institute, 1990; Malcolm, 1991). Given statistics of HIV infection for self-injecting drug using populations and the association between unsafe sexual practices and chemical use, inmates with alcohol and other drug histories clearly are at high risk for HIV infection (Andrus, Fleming, Knox et al., 1989; Hammet, 1989; Harding, 1987). A recent New York State Department of Health study examining HIV seroprevalence of entrants at two correctional sites found, for example, that almost half of all persons entering prison with a history of self-injecting drug use were HIV infected (New York State Department of Health AIDS Institute, 1990).

A number of correctional facilities have developed specific guidelines for the care of those with HIV disease while incarcerated. Of these facilities, some allow for counseling services through community based AIDS organizations (Forbes, 1990). Mental health practitioners available to incarcerated individuals and aware of the complex needs of incarcerated individuals with HIV disease and chemical dependency have the opportunity to have a tremendous impact on the quality of life of this unique population.

This article presents general information on incarcerated individuals with HIV disease, psychosocial issues confronting the inmate with chemical dependency histories and HIV disease, and counseling strategies effective in promoting a "working alliance" between the provider and the incarcerated HIV infected client with a history of past or current use of illicit chemicals.

HIV DISEASE AND THE PRISON SYSTEM

There is a three-tiered system for housing incarcerated populations with the U.S.: the federal system operated by the Federal Bureau of Prisons, the state system, and the local system including county, city, or local jails for short-term incarcerations or detention for inmates awaiting trial (Greenspan, 1989; Vaid, 1987). Currently, over 500,000 men and women are incarcerated in the U.S. Historically and presently, the poor and people of color are incarcerated at numbers disproportionate to the rest of the population (Ryan, 1976; Richan, 1988). Further, the seroprevalence of HIV among incarcerated populations would predictably be higher than the general population based upon statistics of cause for incarceration, percentages of HIV infection for those with self-injecting drug histories, and the association between unsafe sexual practices and chemical use (Vaid, 1987; Stall, 1988).

In order for inmates with HIV disease to receive counseling and/ or advocacy services around HIV infection, a preexisting relationship between a correctional facility and a community-based AIDS education and service organization is required. Even then, counselors who are admitted to a correctional facility may not be viewed as "professionals" but rather as volunteers. Counselors must go through an orientation to the prison, be fingerprinted for a background security check, and have photo-ID cards made before gaining entrance into the facility in the same manner as individuals from outside organizations such as Alcoholics Anonymous. Inmates may learn of the AIDS Service Organization (ASO) while incarcerated, either from other inmates or from educational presentations conducted within the prison setting by ASO educators. They may also have knowledge of the ASO from the community prior to incarceration. Inmates contacting the ASO usually request information, education, and counseling about HIV disease. In all likelihood, the incarcerated individual will be primarily contacting an ASO requesting counseling services knowing that they are HIV infected or upon receiving a diagnosis of AIDS or ARC.

The knowledge of one's HIV status or AIDS diagnosis may be determined either before incarceration or while in custody (Greenspan, 1989). Many correctional facilities employ HIV testing at intake, and it is either offered to inmates who are considered "high-risk" candidates or it is mandated for all inmates (National Prison Project, 1990). The issues around testing for HIV and incarcerated populations are complex. An individual's HIV status/AIDS diagnosis may be known to the administration as part of his or her criminal records. It may have been an issue in prior criminal proceedings, and therefore disclosure to the facility is involuntary. Inmates going through the intake process of a correctional facility may be unfamiliar with administration policy regarding housing, medical care, access to programs, and meals for HIV infected inmates and therefore an individual may self-disclose their HIV status under the presumption or false assumption that such disclosure will benefit their incarceration. At best, an inmate's confidentiality may be compromised once their HIV status is known to prison officials. At worst, an inmate may be segregated from other inmates and placed in an isolation unit under 18-23 hour lock-up, even if asymptomatic, while simultaneously being denied access to other programs such as drug/alcohol treatment if available, education, or recreational options (Lambert, 1990).

Inmates may experience multiple stigmatization around their incarceration and criminal history, their alcohol and other drug histories, and their HIV infection. Corrections officers may use extraordinary precautions such as wearing latex gloves and masks to escort segregated inmates to the infirmary, for example, or to visits with ASO counselors and their attorneys, or to transport inmates to court appearances and outside hospital infectious disease clinic appointments. This may exacerbate an inmate's feelings of isolation and low self-esteem. These complex issues of confidentiality, segregation, and isolation may contribute as well to an increased sense of anxiety and feelings of helplessness in an incarcerated individual and are often the issues that precipitate an inmate seeking counseling services.

Another area that creates distress and heightened anxiety for incarcerated individuals is the availability and quality of health care. Administration policy may be strict regarding the use of medications such as the anti-viral drug AZT (Moore, Hamb, Greenberg, 1990). Inmates may have prior knowledge about or learn that AZT is clinically beneficial while asymptomatic with T-cells of 500, but corrections officials and/or medical staff may only make this drug available to individuals with a diagnosis of AIDS and low T-cell counts. If AZT is prescribed, there may be limited routine monitoring of the effects. According to inmate reports, AZT may not be administered as prescribed but rather in a random manner. In addition, inmates are denied access to major FDA-approved clinical drug trials. Incarcerated PWAs may routinely be transported to area hospital infectious disease clinics where they must wait without appointments to be seen by physicians. Given swelling caseloads at ID clinics, incarcerated PWAs report that they often wait hours to be seen by physicians. It is not uncommon for corrections officers to get tired of waiting, especially if their shift is scheduled to change, and return the inmates to the correctional facility without being seen by a physician. While in the presence of other patients in clinics, they may be shackled in public waiting areas with armed corrections officers wearing masks and gloves, heightening their sense of stigma and humiliation.

For most incarcerated PWAs, medical counseling about treatment options is not routinely provided nor is information in regard to HIV progression, symptomatology, health maintenance, preventative health care, or nutritional counseling. While adequate health care has been defined as a basic human right for incarcerated individuals by the Supreme Court, access to adequate medical care may be limited for the incarcerated PWA (Vaid, 1987). Dietary needs may be disregarded and vitamins are generally not available nor are liquid nutritional supplements for weight gain. Inmates may be seen only in the jail infirmary. The limitations of infirmary medical care make it clearly inadequate for those with HIV disease. Only if their condition becomes critical are they transported to an area hospital. There, they may be treated in a security ward specific to incarcerated populations or mainstreamed throughout the hospital and shackled to existing and available beds with armed corrections officers stationed outside their door.

PSYCHOSOCIAL ISSUES

Chemical dependency issues are of primary concern to many incarcerated individuals. Those with a history of chemical dependency may have feelings of low self-esteem and remorse around past use, particularly if related to their incarceration. Individuals may be arrested when in a period of active use and detoxified while imprisoned. Anguish about drug use may intensify, in addition to the experience of being overwhelmed by incarceration. Suddenly, the incarcerated PWA may be flooded by an awareness of his or her circumstances. The incarcerated PWA may be physically isolated from the rest of the prison population with limited access to information. They may be denied access to drug treatment, even if such programs are available to other inmates, due to segregated housing. They are alone, without a support system, often have limited access to friends, family and loved ones who may have rejected them. Finally, in many instances, incarcerated individuals continue to use illicit psychoactive drugs which are accessible within the prison systems.

Individuals who are incarcerated with a diagnosis of AIDS or HIV spectrum disease have fears about the course of their illness. Foremost is the anguish about dying while incarcerated. For example, it is suggested that incarcerated individuals with HIV disease have a significantly lower life expectancy than non-incarcerated individuals with HIV disease (Gilbert, 1989; Lambert, 1990a). It has been reported in one study in New York that 28% of the deaths attributed to AIDS among inmates were not diagnosed until autopsy (Lambert, 1990b). Typically, there is a preoccupation with death and a heightened realization of the limits imposed upon them by incarceration. Incarcerated PWAs often dwell upon missed opportunities and feelings of not being able to "turn their life around." Depending upon the quantity of time lost due to incarceration and potential loss of their future due to HIV, these feelings must be addressed and reconciled in counseling sessions.

Inmates may have alienated themselves from family members especially if there is a history of alcohol and other drug dependency. At a time when they are particularly in need of familial support, it may not be available to them. Inmates with children, either male or female, who have histories of lengthy incarcerations and alcohol or other drug use often have had little physical or emotional contact with their children. This can be experienced as a tremendous loss; a diagnosis of AIDS heightens this loss. Hope may be shattered that one day things will be different and circumstances will change in a positive manner. Families who may have been involved with an inmate through years of drinking, drugging, and criminal behavior may now reject this family member when their HIV status is learned. Families may blame the individual for becoming HIV infected and also for potentially infecting or exposing other family members to HIV, regardless of mutual risk behaviors. Even though there may be tremendous conflicts within a family system, inmates typically express a longing to reestablish relationships with family members, and counselors can be instrumental in facilitating these contacts.

Incarcerated PWAs with HIV disease report physical abuse and sexual intimidation by fellow prisoners and also by corrections officers. Inmates may be victimized by corrections officers who resent having to physically work with the HIV infected due to a perceived personal risk of exposure to the virus. Other inmates whose HIV status is not known may also ostracize and be aggressive towards the HIV infected incarcerated individual. They are perceived as a legitimate object to direct aggression towards given their status within the prison system.

Another area of major concern for inmates with HIV disease is sexual expression. Sexual behavior between inmates has been well-documented (Wooden and Parker, 1982). However, availability of condoms and dental dams is severely limited and they may be considered contraband by prison administration which makes practicing safer sex virtually impossible among inmates. Guilt and shame are common reactions among inmates who are aware of their HIV infection and who engage in unsafe sexual practices.

Given the physical setting of a correctional facility and a diagnosis of AIDS, most inmates have difficulty dealing with their feelings and circumstances. For an individual who until recently has also been using mood-altering chemicals or who continues to use such substances while incarcerated, the ability to cope is even more complex and limited. Non-chemically induced coping strategies may be less developed. Support systems are often limited or nonexistent. There may be greater internal turmoil in terms of guilt and shame over past behaviors. Because of these issues, adjustment to living with HIV is further complicated for the HIV infected inmate with a chemical dependency history.

COUNSELING STRATEGIES

The availability of counseling may be limited due to the lack of service provided to inmates by community-based ASOs. Some ASOs offer services to incarcerated populations, some do not. If services exist, there should be a policy of accepting collect phone calls from incarcerated PWAs. If services are provided, workers knowledgeable about AIDS may still lack knowledge or exposure to the specific issues of incarcerated populations with histories of chemical dependency. Therefore, counselors need to familiarize themselves with the issues that pertain to this population. Anyone attempting to work with this population also needs to assess their own feelings and projections around incarcerated individuals and individuals with chemical dependency histories. AIDS service organizations need to sensitize their staff to a number of issues inherent in working with incarcerated populations, including multiculturalism, chemical dependency, racism, and historically disenfranchised populations.

For the counselor, the experience of entering a correctional facility may by initially intimidating. The counselor can not, however, allow these feelings to overwhelm him or her and must be certain never to be judgmental, blaming, or oversolicitous. Most importantly, the counselor must express to the incarcerated HIV client with a chemical use history that despite unacceptable criminal behavior, he or she is a worthwhile human being. Clients need to be aware of the parameters of the relationship in terms of what the contact is about, the goals of the treatment, length of the relationship, and counselor time availability. The client needs to be aware of the limitations imposed upon the counselor by the facility. These may include inconsistencies in meeting times due to lack of controls over the environment. Officers may not bring inmates to visitation rooms as scheduled. Incarcerated PWAs may be sent to another activity at a counselor's prescheduled meeting time. Inmates may be punished overtly or covertly and may be in lockup. Counseling parameters must focus on the counseling relationship and goals of treatment rather than on the client's legal case. For example, either out of desperation or an attempt to manipulate the counselor, the inmate may wish to encourage involvement with a legal case beyond the scope, influence, or expertise of the counselor. A client should be encouraged to express his or her feelings and discuss issues around an impending legal cases. But the counselor needs to remember that they are not there in the role of legal consultant.

Incarcerated individuals have understandable skepticism regarding trusting "professionals." In order to build a good counseling relationship the inmate needs to know that this counselor/client relationship is governed by the laws of confidentiality. The inmate will need to be reassured that none of the information discussed will be shared within or outside the correctional facility.

Counselors working with incarcerated individuals can expect to realistically provide education about HIV disease, symptomatology, HIV progression, available treatment options, and fundamental dietary and nutritional care. Discussions about safer sex practices need to be integrated into counseling (Shernoff, 1988), as does information about the safer injection of drugs and sterilization of injection equipment. Further, inmates need to be informed about the link between ongoing active substance use and HIV progression, resultant consequences, impaired immune system functioning and educated about the disease concept of chemical dependency. The relationship between the increased likelihood of engaging in unsafe behaviors while under the influence of mood-altering substances should be emphasized.

The counselor needs to be consistent and available within the limitations imposed by the correctional facility. The counselor represents a bridge between the prison and the outside world, providing information that might not otherwise exist. A counselor should also refer inmates where appropriate to 12-step programs such as

AA or NA, if they exist within the correctional facility. If there are not AA or NA meetings going on within the prison, the counselor would be providing an important service by advocating with the prison administration to allow such meetings to be conducted.

Counselors need to monitor their expectations regarding the outcome of counseling with this population. Even when a good relationship between the inmate-client and counselor exists, there may be only limited resolution of internal conflicts and distress. The counselor can assist the inmate in making life more tolerable and in developing a plan for the future. Often, this requires that the counselor not join with the incarcerated PWAs false hopes and unrealistic expectations of release. Thus, much of the focus of counseling sessions needs to be on the context of the client's present life circumstances and on ways of maximizing the quality of the incarcerated individual's life and obtaining satisfactions within the confines of prison.

The education provided about HIV-related illnesses and chemical dependency reduces self-blame and stigma and teaches inmates that they are not at fault for these diseases. Education can be empowering, suggesting that they can pro-actively become involved in their health management. This is particularly salient for individuals with a chemical dependency history because it can become a motivating factor to maintain abstinence while incarcerated and upon release. Social support for the incarcerated PWA allows for social skill development in a drug-free relationship. A counselor can help in this phase, which is important if and when the inmate is released from prison. The counselor may be the only positive influence to sustain the inmate's chemical dependency abstinence and the promotion of self-worth, particularly if an inmate is in an isolation unit with no access to treatment or to ongoing institutional AA meetings.

CASE STUDY

James is a 34 year-old black male who contacted an ASO by making a collect call from a county jail. He stated that he learned of available counseling services from other inmates and wanted to become a client. Since all counselors had access to the correctional facility, an appointment was made for an intake and assessment to determine his need for services. The only time made available for an intake by the correctional facility was during regular visiting hours. As a result, the intake was conducted in a crowded, open visitation room at a time when all inmates can receive visits from family and friends.

During the intake, James revealed that he thought he had a diagnosis of AIDS, wasn't completely certain about whether or not he had AIDS though he had tested HIV positive. He also revealed an extensive alcohol and drug history, including a history of self-injecting drug use that was directly related to his current incarceration. He stated he believed the route of transmission of HIV was from drug use through shared injection equipment. He stated that he had requested an HIV antibody test at the jail upon intake when it was offered to him. Upon receiving his test results, he was housed in a segregation block in 18 hour lockup with other inmates who were known to be HIV infected or who had AIDS.

His stated needs were for information about AIDS and counseling to deal with his fears of an unknown future. He stated that he had been unfamiliar with the policy of segregation of HIV infected inmates, and had he known, would not have chosen to be tested. After the intake was processed, James was assigned a counselor and a contract was established for short-term counseling. James initially focused on his lack of knowledge about whether or not he had AIDS. He was furnished information about HIV disease progression, symptomatology, and available treatment options. James reported that during his previous incarceration at a state facility, he had been hospitalized for pneumonia and then released on parole shortly thereafter. He did not know if his pneumonia was bacterial or PCP. James agreed to sign a consent form to send for his medical records from the state correctional facility.

James expressed a great deal of anxiety about the uncertainty of his diagnosis. He reported questioning the medical staff at the jail infirmary but had received ambiguous responses. He had previously been taken to the county medical center's infectious disease clinic for blood work but as yet had not been given any information about the results and was not currently receiving any medications.

As a result of information supplied to James in counseling, he became more knowledgeable about HIV disease and treatments. He became aggressive and empowered regarding his health care and thus more demanding of the medical staff in the infirmary about their course of treatment. He started making requests in writing for copies of his blood work, specifically regarding his T-4 cell counts. He was frustrated when these reports were not forthcoming from the infirmary. Signed consent forms were obtained for the counselor to send for medical information from the county medical center. When the medical records were received by the ASO, they revealed that only routine blood tests had been taken, and T-cell tests had not been done. This information was conveyed to James, who then requested through the infirmary to the physician at the county medical center that these tests be performed. He received an appointment for six weeks later at the infectious disease clinic. He then began a period of waiting, not only for the appointment but also for the results. Ultimately, tests revealed a low T-cell count, and James was placed on AZT.

James's requests for information about HIV infection resulted in reducing his feelings of uncertainty. The fact that James let both the prison and county medical personnel know that he had an assigned counselor from an outside organization probably contributed to his receiving better care.

Counseling also began to focus on James's substance abuse. After being paroled back into the community from the state prison, he had resumed using illicit drugs and alcohol. He was rearrested and charged with driving a stolen car and with possession of illegal drugs, for which he was currently incarcerated in the county jail while awaiting hearings. He stated that he had been in a blackout at the time he was arrested and could only vaguely recall the specifics of the event. He claimed that it was while he was still under the influence of alcohol and illicit drugs that he was asked if he wanted an HIV test and didn't remember pretest counseling when he consented.

The counselor assisted James in linking his use of drugs with his present circumstances. The consequences of his illicit drug use in terms of imprisonment, HIV status and loss of time became the focus of sessions rather than the inappropriateness of how he became aware of his HIV infection. As the relationship between chemical use and James's present circumstances became established, James's emotional distress escalated, and he was able to express anguish, grief, and remorse.

James shared with the counselor that he was using drugs while in prison when they were available. Sessions then focused on helping James consider the consequences of his present drug use, including the potential increased HIV symptomatology and possible loss of the counseling relationship as a consequence of using. The counselor offered James an alternative to using drugs by suggesting he keep a journal and write down his feelings as if the counselor were available. This was especially important because he was housed in an isolation unit and had no access to the drug treatment program available to other inmates within the system whose HIV status wasn't known. AA meetings within the prison were also denied to him because of his HIV status. The journal became a symbol of support and connectedness to the counselor. In addition, it allowed for James to manage his feelings and increased his ability to cope with his circumstances. The journal effectively reduced James's focus on relapsing into active drug use.

James became increasingly concerned about the quality of care for himself and others with HIV disease in the facility where he was incarcerated. The counselor encouraged James to advocate for himself and others about this issue. He discussed the need for more contact among the other PWAs and wrote a letter to the administration requesting a support group, which did begin as a direct result of James's efforts. His ability to organize and follow through with a plan of action was reinforced by the counselor.

As the counseling relationship unfolded, James went from feeling hopeless and destitute to realizing that he had the potential to turn his life around and gain satisfaction. The experience of having a group formed as a result of his letter to the prison administration gave James evidence that he could affect his circumstances. This led to discussions of future activity and the possibility of his eventual release from prison. James had a desire to become a role model in his community upon release from prison, particularly to other young men of color at risk for HIV disease. This was supported by the counselor as a component of aftercare planning. In addition, James was encouraged to continue to engage in counseling services either while incarcerated, depending on the outcome of his criminal case, or once released and to also involve himself in AA and NA.

CONCLUSION

The incarcerated individual with HIV disease and chemical dependency faces a multiplicity of issues as a function of imprisonment, medical status, and chemical use history. The complexity of concerns may be overwhelming to clients and counselors alike. This paper has recommended a general plan for counselor intervention. The initial focus of intervention on education can serve to establish the counselor's expertise and value to the client, express the counselor's warmth and nonjudgmental regard, and set the stage for later interventions of social and emotional support. Information allows for the beginning of a counseling relationship, reduces anxiety, and empowers the client. The provision of counseling services to the incarcerated individual with HIV disease and a history of chemical dependency is important both individually and socially. Clients who receive counseling services while incarcerated may experience reduced distress and improved health simply as a function of social support. Linkages between community-based AIDS service organizations and the prisons allow for a continuity of care in the community should incarcerated clients be released. This is significant in terms of prevention of future criminal behavior, relapse into alcohol and other drug use and unsafe sexual practices, and accessing appropriate medical care with a population who may otherwise be reluctant to engage in services.

Providing counseling to incarcerated individuals with HIV disease and a history of chemical dependency is both challenging and rewarding. Perhaps the most fulfilling aspect of the work is impacting upon the lives of clients so desperately in need of care, concern, and support.

REFERENCES

Andrus, J. K., Fleming, D. W., Knox, C., McAlister, R.O., Skeels, M. R., Conrad, R. E., Horan, J. M., and Foster, L. R. (1989). "HIV testing in prisoners: is mandatory testing mandatory?" *American Journal of Public Health*, 79(7), 840-842.

Forbes, A. (1990). "Preventing AIDS and serving people with AIDS 'on the inside.'" *The Exchange* (in press.)

Foucault, M. (1977). *Discipline and Punish: The Birth of The Prison*. New York: Vintage Books.

Gilbert, D. (1989). "Educating prisoners," *Focus, A Guide to AIDS Research and Counseling*, 4(6), 3.

Greenspan, J. (1988). "NPP gathers statistics on AIDS in prison." *National Prison Project Journal*, 16, 5-8.

Greenspan, J. (1989). "HIV infection among prisoners." *Focus*, 4 (6), 1-2.

Hammet, T. M. (1989). *Update 1988: AIDS in Correctional Facilities*. Washington, D.C.: National Institute of Justice, 27.

Harding, T. W. (1987). "AIDS in prison." *Lancet*, 2(8570), 1260-1263.

Lambert, B. (1990). "Prisons criticized on AIDS programs."*The New York Times*, August 19, 16.

Lambert, B. (1990). "Suit faults AIDS care in New York prisons." *The New York Times*, March 8, B3.

Malcolm, A (1991). "More cells for more prisoners, but to what end?" *The New York Times*, January 18, B16.

Moore, L., Hamb, A., Greenberg, R. (1990). "Medical and psychological issues in HIV/AIDS and health concerns for incarcerated populations." Panel discussion at the National Lesbian and Gay Health Conference and AIDS Forum. Washington, D.C.

National Commission on AIDS. (1991). *Report on HIV Disease in Correctional Facilities*, Washington, D.C.

National Prison Project (1990). *AIDS in Prison Bibliography*. Washington, D.C.

New York State Department of Health AIDS Institute. (1990). "Management of HIV infection in New York State prisons," *Focus on AIDS in New York State*, 2(1), 1-3.

Richan, W. C. (1988). *Beyond altruism: social welfare policy in American society*. New York: The Haworth Press, Inc.

Ryan, W. (1976). *Blaming the victim*. New York: Vintage Books.

Shernoff, M. (1988). "Integrating safer-sex counseling into social work practice," *Social Casework*, 69(6), 334-339.

Stall, R. (1988). "The Prevention of HIV infection associated with drug and alcohol use during sexual activity," in L. Siegel, (Ed). *AIDS and Substance Abuse*, New York: Harrington Park Press, 73-88.

Vaid, U. (1987). "Prisoners." In H. L. Dalton and S. Burrow, (Eds.) *AIDS and the Law*. New Haven: Yale University Press, 235-250.

Wooden, W. & Parker, J. (1982). *Men behind bars. sexual exploitation in prison*. New York and London, Plenum Press.

The Use of Outpatient Psychotherapy with Chemically Dependent HIV Infected Individuals

Michele Fontaine, MA

Whenever an individual who is chemically dependent learns that he or she is infected with HIV, they are immediately faced with additional and new-life stressors. Not only does this person have to cope with all of the issues surrounding their addiction, but in addition they are faced with the challenges inherent in adjusting to living with HIV infection and potentially the life threatening condition of full-blown AIDS. There are very limited services available for a chemically dependent HIV infected individual, particularly if he or she is actively using drugs. Various outpatient psychotherapy clinics offer services for this special population, but only if the individual has had some recovery time. When someone who is chemically dependent learns that he or she is HIV positive, this often acts as a catalyst for the person to cope the best way they have learned, namely by using drugs. Outpatient psychotherapy, by itself, cannot provide enough support and treatment for a person who is both chemically dependent and HIV infected, especially if the individual is actively using drugs. However, outpatient psychosocial services can add an important component of care within a whole array of treatment by providing a supplemental support system for a client that is already engaged in various other support systems or by becoming the sole support system for an isolated individual.

What follows is a description of work conducted in the AIDS Mental Health Project of Greenwich House Counseling Center. Located in Manhattan, Greenwich House is a multimodality agency specializing in the outpatient treatment of people who have a history of abusing alcohol and/or drugs.

The AIDS Mental Health Project has been in existence since March, 1988. The basic mission of the project is to provide outpatient psychotherapy to HIV infected chemical abusers who are either actively using or are in recovery. The project has also been designed to work with family members and all significant others of this population. Since the project's inception, we have run three successful support groups with a fourth one currently being organized. Our primary catchment area is Greenwich Village and Chelsea on the lower west side of Manhattan, yet we have admitted individuals from all over the Greater New York City metropolitan area and from New Jersey. Two of the most innovative and significant aspects of the project have been the fact that we admit active users and that we have a highly specialized staff who is comfortable working with this population.

A very specific drug and treatment history is taken at intake during which the therapist seeks to learn the following: when was each drug and/or alcohol first used; has the client ever experienced seizures, overdoses or blackouts; has the client had any recovery time and are they using any other support systems; is the client currently using and if so, how much and how often; and finally, what has been the client's drug of choice (in the past or currently) and why. In addition to the drug history, a psychodynamic assessment of the client is completed that includes an assessment of his or her mental status.

Obviously, therapeutic approaches when working with a recovering chemically dependent individual and a person who is actively using drugs are totally different. A conventional outpatient model of psychotherapy with an individual who has been exposed to HIV or is symptomatic with AIDS and has a history of chemical dependence yet is drug free is more applicable than with an individual who is not drug free. Often the client is seen two times a week for individual sessions and is given the option of joining a support group in addition to individual treatment.

There are two primary goals of treatment with HIV positive clients who have been "clean and dry." The first goal is to help the client remain free of drugs and/or alcohol. Concurrent with this is the goal of providing the clients with a safe place to discuss their growing anxiety and or depression as related to concerns about the progression of their illness and possible death.

Once the psychodynamic assessment is completed the therapist is usually able to anticipate what situations may trigger signals that place the client at risk for relapsing into active use. The therapist points these out to the client in an attempt to build in nondrug using responses to the inevitable stressors that arise from both being in recovery and living with HIV infection. In general the therapeutic approach is a combination of behavioral and self-psychological/ego supportive approaches when working with the client's growing anxiety over his/her current health status or future deterioration.

Our staff takes a totally different approach when working with an individual who is actively using drugs and/or alcohol. The one firm condition of being seen by a therapist in this program that the clients are informed of during the initial session is that they can't come to sessions under the influence of either alcohol or drugs. If clients persist in arriving for sessions high, in order to continue to be a client they must have a medical detoxification and must begin to attend an appropriate twelve-step program. In addition, clients who continue to actively use drugs or alcohol are referred to the agency's day treatment program and therapy groups that specifically focus on chronic alcohol and/or drug use. Overall, clients are treated in both a structured, confrontive way as well as in a supportive way with the goal being to regain some stability.

Of all the clients seen at the Project, individuals who continue to use drugs and/or alcohol while wishing to access services are undoubtedly the most frustrating to treat in an outpatient setting. This type of client is very taxing to all staff as they are constantly testing how much they can get away with without being terminated from the program. However, 50% of all active users who have applied to the Project have been retained in treatment during which periods of relapse and/or bingeing as well as some periods of stability are the norm.

Three case studies will be presented in which each person's psychosocial history will be given, followed by a description of the outpatient psychotherapy.

Alan was first admitted into the project in November, 1988. He is a forty year-old, Caucasian, bisexual male. He began using glue at age ten, intravenous heroin at eleven, alcohol and barbiturates at twelve, intravenous crystal methedrine at thirteen, and intravenous cocaine as well. His drug of choice has been intravenously administered crystal methedrine and cocaine.

Alan was diagnosed HIV positive in September 1987. His presenting issue was severe depression with possible suicidal ideation as a combined reaction to both his own health status and the death of his lover from AIDS two months before he sought admission to our program. At the time of intake, he was sharing an apartment with another man. He had a history of psychiatric hospitalizations in state hospitals from ages thirteen through sixteen and a history of attempted suicide by using drugs, the most recent attempt having been one month prior to the death of his lover.

Alan described his family as intact, with four siblings, but very dysfunctional with an active alcoholic father who had been physically abusive. At the time of Alan's intake one of his brother's had an AIDS diagnosis and the other was an addict living in Florida. Alan was "given away" at age eleven to an older man, at which point he was sexually abused by his guardian. Contact with his family had recently resumed after a long period of noncommunication.

Alan described his interpersonal skills as quite sophisticated except for periodic bouts of isolating. Vocationally, he accumulated various clerical skills while in the Marine Corps but was most interested in making a living cooking. At intake he was unemployed and on Public Assistance. Prior to learning that he was infected with HIV, Alan had been very sexually active with a large number of different partners. Aside from periodic attendance at AA meetings, Alan had had no treatment for his drug use prior to contacting Greenwich House. By attending AA, Alan had one period of seven and a half years when he was completely alcohol free.

Two years after intake, Alan is being seen two times per week for individual psychotherapy. He has had five relapses since admission, during which he used cocaine intravenously, and one relapse, during which he used crack. He had also had himself admitted to an inpatient psychiatric service twice, once in the Spring of 1989, and again, in January 1990. Both hospitalizations were in response to severe depression and concurrent cocaine abuse. During the course of treatment this client has attended NA for two different periods of time, the longest period lasting approximately eight and a half months. Since initially presenting at our agency, his HIV condition has progressed so that he is currently mildly symptomatic. In addition, during one four month period, Alan's best friend and his brother both died from AIDS, and his mother also died. Alan's capacity for insight into his own behavior has developed to such an extent that he has been able to understand that he uses drugs as a direct response to the pain he felt from the losses he sustained. Rather than tolerate the feeling of emptiness and subsequent depression, he attempted to numb himself by using drugs. When the drug use failed to shut off his uncomfortable feelings, he requested psychiatric hospitalization in an effort to try and learn how to cope with everything that was causing stress in his life. After two years of therapy he has just begun to express anxieties about getting sick from HIV and possibly dying from AIDS like his lover, his brother, and his close friend.

During the course of treatment Alan also became homeless. This situation was rectified when he was admitted to a supportive housing facility for persons with AIDS. Most of his relapses were due to his inability to tolerate feeling increasingly depressed as he became progressively symptomatic and to his difficulty in openly mourning his losses. He has never come to sessions high and always expressed a motivation to stay clean.

Therapeutic approaches have been behavioral and ego supportive. For the first year of treatment, sessions were mostly crisis intervention in response to his feeling overwhelmed, depressed, or unable to manage the concrete tasks relating to his health status. Thus sessions were often concrete "trouble shooting" counseling sessions that were problem-solving oriented. This approach helped the client to develop trust in the therapist, as well as to deal with a variety of life situations that he was having difficulty managing, including health maintenance issues pertaining to his physical condition.

Early in treatment, Alan's drug use was often out of control and as a result of that, the other areas in his life were chaotic and often unattended to. This obviously helped contribute to a deterioration of his physical condition since during periods of active drug use, eating well ceased to be a priority for him. Sessions were primarily spent looking at specific behaviors before and during the relapses in an attempt to teach him to recognize the early warning signs of an impending relapse and how to interrupt the progression towards using drugs by reaching out to staff or people in NA. The goals of working in this way were to help him avoid relying on drugs as a sole coping mechanism and to help him gain some stability in his life.

Since periods of active drug use have lessened in duration and frequency, the content of sessions has been more ego supportive. Alan's denial about being infected with HIV has lessened as his drug use has diminished. Sessions have focused on quality of life issues such as relationships and expanding his support systems. Alan has also begun to talk directly about his fears of physically deteriorating and dying. One of the therapist's goals has been to encourage Alan to voice his fears and concerns about his health and validate the normalcy of these feelings. In addition, the therapist has been urging Alan to express his rage and sadness about the deaths of so many people he has loved.

In response to his severe ongoing depression, Alan was referred for a psychiatric evaluation, which resulted in his being prescribed Prozac which helped ameliorate some of the symptoms of the depression. It has only been after the most severe symptoms of his depression abated as a result of the medication that he has been able to freely discuss the painful material described above. It seems clear that Alan is benefiting from a maintenance dose of Prozac, and therapy provides a place to regularly support his taking the medication as prescribed.

He has used treatment and referrals to outside community-based supports effectively. The primary focus of treatment at the time of this writing is to help him find work or vocational training, which tends to provide a foundation around which he has stabilized himself in the past. In addition, as his physical condition worsens, therapy can provide him with a place to discuss all of his feelings relating to his changing health status in a supportive and safe environment. Teaching Alan to identify and recognize "relapse triggers" before he acts out on them also remains a focus of treatment.

Barry is a thirty-one year-old, Caucasian, homosexual male, who was first seen in March, 1989. He began using alcohol at age ten, intravenous speed at fourteen, and intravenous heroin at sixteen. After his parents died when he was nineteen, he began to use cocaine intravenously multiple times daily and Valium tablets as well, becoming addicted to both. His drugs of choice have been intravenous heroin and cocaine. Barry was an active intravenous drug user for most of his early adulthood. His only serious attempt at becoming drug free was an inpatient detox he admitted himself to. Barry was referred to our project by a worker from this detox.

Barry learned he was HIV positive in 1986 and at the time of intake had not had any medical follow up regarding his condition. His presenting issues for therapy were his addiction, maintaining sobriety, and learning to cope with his HIV diagnosis. At intake, he was living with a friend waiting placement in supportive housing for people with AIDS. Most of his support network at this time was through twelve-step programs that he had begun during detox. He also reported having had numerous contacts with psychiatrists and psychologists.

He grew up in the southern United States in an intact and dysfunctional family. His father was an alcoholic, and his mother abused prescription drugs. He reported being very close to his older sister and having a half brother from his father's second marriage, with whom he was not close. Barry was sexually abused by male cousins when he was a child from age six through eleven. Initially, he was gang raped and continued to be abused on and off for several years. He knew he was gay at age thirteen and prostituted from age fourteen to twenty-eight. He attributed his drug and alcohol use to the environment he grew up in.

His parents divorced when he was ten, and both parents died within two weeks of each other. After the death of his parents, Barry bonded with his sister who was addicted to drugs and increased his intake of drugs heavily.

He described often feeling inhibited and insecure about his interpersonal skills. He completed a GED and has had no significant employment history. He has indicated an interest in acting and cooking. Barry has been drug free since he started attending 12-Step meetings in January 1989. He has been in a relationship with another HIV infected man since the summer of 1990 and currently is living with his lover in their own apartment. Barry is hoping to be off welfare next year. He has had increasingly more symptoms of HIV related illnesses but is medically stable.

At the time of this writing Barry is being seen once a week for individual psychotherapy, and the main issue in treatment revolves around his ambivalence regarding intimacy in his life and the new relationship resulting in lessened isolation, all within the context of being infected with HIV. In addition, at about the same time Barry moved in with his new lover, he began to discuss a desire to control his sexual compulsivity which started to surface, addictively, after he began his current relationship indicating ambivalence and discomfort about the closeness and intimacy this relationship provides. His sexual behavior outside the relationship also serves to create some emotional distance from his new lover. Fears about his lover abandoning him by dying from AIDS have occasionally begun to be discussed during therapy sessions. Due to his sobriety, the clinician has been in a position to use both ego-supportive and some ego-modifying techniques.

Barry's old behaviors, beyond his chemical dependency, have been a constant area of discussion, namely his sexual acting out. The therapist has looked at the linkages of this sexual behavior with the client's fears of intimacy—fears that preceded his diagnosis and have escalated since diagnosis. The therapist has attempted to modify these behaviors by looking at their roots and at current catalysts, such as an HIV diagnosis. Throughout this modifying process, the therapist has also remained supportive and not at all judgmental about the various behaviors that Barry is discussing during treatment.

Connie is a forty year-old, Caucasian, lesbian who was first seen in August, 1989. She began using alcohol and marijuana in early adolescence and continued until age twenty-four. At that time, she began using intravenous cocaine until the age of thirty. At thirty, she started using intravenous heroin with other substances until age thirty-two. She entered a methadone program and detoxed from methadone between the ages of thirty-two and thirty-four. At intake, she had been clean for four years. Her drugs of choice had been intravenous heroin and cocaine.

Connie was diagnosed as having progressive symptoms of HIV illness in October 1988. Her presenting issue was an escalating conflict with her lover of eighteen months who was not infected with HIV. She felt that the relationship was deteriorating and that she needed help with her communication skills. Initially treatment consisted of couples' therapy. At intake, the couple was living together. Connie's lover and family were her only sources of emotional support.

Connie has a history of psychiatric treatment, beginning at age nineteen when she was hospitalized for forty days supposedly for a Stelazine reaction. Her parents divorced when Connie was six, and she grew up with her mother and sister. She reported having strong social skills, which she said improved during her sobriety. She obtained an associates degree in paralegal services and at intake was working as a paralegal.

She identified as heterosexual until the age of twenty-four but now considers herself to be a lesbian. She was sexually abused at age eleven by an uncle. She attributed her substance abuse to her environment and peer pressure as well as to her first lesbian lover who was an intravenous heroin user. Yet what appears clear is that this woman has a long history of depression beginning in childhood, exacerbated by being sexually abused, and that drug use was the only option she possessed to ameliorate these feelings.

Currently, Connie is being seen individually, with the couples' therapy having ended three months into treatment. Her lover moved out in January, 1990. This precipitated a serious ongoing depression that has not resolved as of this writing. Shortly after Connie's lover moved out, Connie was diagnosed with full-blown AIDS. The combined stressors of the end of her relationship, diagnosis of AIDS and the unremitting depression caused Connie to relapse into active intravenous heroin and cocaine use shortly after her diagnosis. Several months after being diagnosed with AIDS, a psychiatric evaluation resulted in her being prescribed Sinequan and BusPar which helped moderate some of the symptoms of her depression, yet Connie continued to self-medicate with heroin and cocaine until she was informed that she had to either be medically detoxed from heroin and cocaine or have her treatment ended at the Project. In December of 1990 she agreed to enter a detox program.

During sessions, Connie would obsess over her lost lover as well as ruminate over her deteriorating health. Yet treatment has not really progressed since Connie continues to act impulsively by using drugs. Her depression and anxiety become compounded by her self-destructive behaviors. Her life, mental status, and emotional state have not significantly improved as a result of attending therapy.

Initially, confrontive and cognitive approaches worked well with Connie, helping her to control her urges to use drugs. As her life became more chaotic as a result of her relationship ending, her escalating drug use, and deteriorating health, she has demanded a considerable amount of attention from the therapists who have been working with her. It has become clear that insight-oriented and analytic approaches to therapy have not worked well with this client. She has responded best to a very structured treatment plan that provides her with external structures that make her ever escalating anxiety and depression bearable without needing to resort to drugs. At the time of this writing, some of the treatment structures include multiple therapeutic contacts weekly, even if for a brief period of time, in addition to urging her to attend twelve step program meetings on a daily basis. Future goals remain concrete as opposed to intrapsychic such as helping her remain drug free in a supportive and caring environment.

There are some common themes in treating the three people described above in an outpatient mental health setting and most active drug using individuals who are infected with HIV. The first is the anxiety and/or depression that accompanies the client's deteriorating health status and the overwhelming urges on the part of these clients to numb themselves to these feelings by using drugs. The second issue is the impact of a minimal to moderate level of vocational skills on the client's self-esteem and upon efforts to be economically self-supporting. Clients who continue to actively use drugs have a high degree of ambivalence about attending treatment. This results in inconsistent contacts with the Project. Almost all of the Project's clients have a strong tendency to isolate, which further contributes to the irregularity of attending treatment sessions. Isolation has played a key role in all of the above described clients' lives and has probably been the most common, repeating theme seen in the clinic.

Each of these clients had underlying psychiatric symptoms that predated the onset of their drug use and certainly predated their diagnosis with HIV, and both drug use and the HIV condition exacerbate symptoms like depression and anxiety. An interdisciplinary approach that includes psychiatric evaluation and medication is almost always indicated for these clients. Yet for many substance abuse professionals, an understandable dilemma arises from prescribing psychotropic drugs to people who have a history of or who are currently abusing drugs.

The issue of homelessness and its effects upon clients who are both chemically dependent and infected with HIV is a stressor that has a definite impact upon ongoing treatment. For undomiciled clients who have to spend hours each day trying to find a warm and safe place to spend the night, medical or therapy appointments may simply not be as much of a priority as eating, having a shower, and a bed to sleep in. Thus, it is not always safe to interpret one of these client's missing a session as simply being resistance to treatment. He or she may not have money for transportation to the agency. The effects of homelessness upon an individual with a chronic, debilitating, life threatening illness like HIV has to be looked at realistically when seeking to provide psychosocial supports to this population.

The relapse patterns described above are fairly typical for many of the clients who are or who have been in treatment at the Project. Alan and Connie's relapses have usually occurred as a direct result of increased symptomatology from the HIV, difficulties with relationships due in part to being infected, and increased depression when diagnosed with a new opportunistic infection. Barry has been drug free since admission nearly two years ago and attributes this to his increased sense of both self-esteem and empowerment that are directly connected to his doing extensive, voluntary work in local AIDS service organizations. In addition Barry reports having been terrified by the way his life had completely fallen apart when he was "bottoming out." Also the thought that he had full-blown AIDS motivated him to remain drug and alcohol free.

In closing, it is safe to say that outpatient psychotherapy for an active or recovering chemically dependent individual can often provide an added support system for an individual that has few avenues for support. The combination of isolation and depression are normal for most people who have come to rely upon drugs and/or alcohol. When this same population has to deal with issues surrounding HIV illness, depression and the tendency to isolate escalate. The potential to relapse then becomes quite strong and the need for the therapist to provide structure and support for clients become even more necessary.

The need for more outpatient services willing to serve individuals who are still actively using drugs who are also coping with HIV is overwhelming. This special, very underserved, and exceptionally needy population requires this kind of mental health service in addition to other clinical services in order to obtain some stability in their lives from both their addiction and their medical condition.

Residential Treatment
for Chemically Dependent
Clients with HIV

Melvin I. Pohl, MD

There are certain specific areas that arise in a residential treatment setting when treating the chemically dependent HIV positive client (CDHC). In this article, residential treatment refers to a twenty-eight to thirty-five day program. The goals of such programs are abstinence from mood-altering chemicals and connection with a Twelve-Step Program in order to have a lifelong recovery from the disease of chemical dependency. The quality of sobriety is therefore based on the modification of stressors and coming to grips with people, places, and things that do not meet the client's satisfaction. In a treatment setting such as this, HIV infection and AIDS are major life obstacles that requires special attention. I will use "HIV" as shorthand for all HIV infection, whether symptomatic, asymptomatic, or full blown AIDS.

HIV infection is truly an exacerbating phenomenon for chemically dependent clients undergoing entering residential treatment. There are many reasons why this is so: (1) Many HIV positive clients believe in the myth that being HIV positive signals death. CDHCs often suffer from more intense depression and hopelessness than non-HIV positive clients and often ask, "Why get sober just to die from AIDS?" (2) Many people with HIV infection are convinced that they will never be able to find a loving relationship that has meaning. (3) The diagnosis of HIV infection usually intensifies the guilt and shame that most chemically dependent patients experience both about their substance abuse and past sexual behaviors. (4) A client's HIV infection makes him or her "different" from the general client population, underscoring the sense of uniqueness that most chemically dependent people experience. (5) CDHCs may have symptoms that lead a physician to prescribe mood-altering chemicals, which would be contraindicated for most chemically dependent clients in recovery. (6) Many chemically dependent clients entering a residential program are estranged from their family of origin due to their sexual orientation (if lesbian or gay) or their drug-using behavior. HIV infection complicates the process of family reconciliation. (7) CDHCs often have medical needs that exceed those of other chemically dependent clients making greater demands on staff and the facility. (8) The diagnosis of HIV and the clients' emotional responses to this often seem so urgent that these issues can become the primary focus in the treatment process, thus becoming a distraction from the tasks essential for the work of early recovery from chemical dependence.

Obviously the issues involved in working with clients with HIV make the clinician's job more complicated. The task of the counselor is to be familiar with and acknowledge the differences for CDHCs while maintaining a focus on recovery from chemical dependence by developing a treatment plan specific to the individual client.

Residential treatment is divided into three phases: assessment and detoxification, treatment planning, and continuing care. The following discussion will contrast treatment for CDHCs and treatment for the general population of chemically dependent clients.

ASSESSMENT

The assessment process includes evaluating the client's chemical use history and consequences of use (physical, psychological, interpersonal, employment, financial, and spiritual). A chemical dependency professional also needs to assess a client's willingness and motivation to achieve and maintain sobriety. This work is done by evaluating past attempts at sobriety, including a history of prior treatment. Medical and psychiatric complications need to be evaluated thoroughly.

In order to meet criteria for admission to a residential setting, a client must be in need of round-the-clock monitoring, structure, and support while not being too medically or psychiatrically disabled to participate in an active-treatment program.

When evaluating the admission of a CDHC, it is important to thoroughly assess the medical and psychological effects of the client's HIV infection. Basic information including actual diagnosis, length of time with the diagnosis, symptoms, history of opportunistic infections, and treatment are essential in the early assessment phase. Also, the client's need for medical care must be matched to the ability of the facility to provide such care (e.g., medication administration, including the need for pentamidine by inhalation, diagnostic testing, and the need for experimental drugs). An assessment of the client's cognitive abilities must be made. Residential treatment requires some amount of cognitive clarity. Most chemically dependent people who are actively using have some impairment of cognition. It is therefore important to assess the combined effect of drug use and HIV infection on a client's ability to participate intellectually in the treatment program.

Next, it is important to assess how a client's HIV infection is interacting with his or her use of mood-altering chemicals on an emotional level. It is not uncommon for the diagnosis of HIV or the progression of the illness into a symptomatic state to cause relapse into use of drugs or alcohol. Is the client in need of prescribed mood-altering drugs to treat a condition associated with the HIV infection (e.g., reactive or organic depression, severe anxiety, or painful neuropathy)? Many clients as part of their treatment for HIV infection become addicted to anxiolytic drugs, sleeping medications, and pain relievers. Medical personnel at residential facilities must be familiar with both HIV infection and chemical dependency in order to evaluate and differentiate drugs of abuse from drugs that are essential for symptom control. This line is often blurred by a client's emotional response to their HIV infection and must be assessed carefully as clients may use HIV related symptomatology in an effort to manipulate staff or obtain drugs that their condition does not require.

It is important to assess a client's level of depression and potential for suicide. Many CDHCs hit "bottom" hard and are even more at risk for suicidal thoughts and gestures, if not actual attempts. If a client is judged to be suicidal, appropriate monitoring and intervention must be instituted.

A client's motivation is often the best indicator of her/his ability to maintain sobriety. According to the *Alcoholics Anonymous* text, those who get well are "willing to go to any lengths" "since half measures availed us nothing." Assessment of motivation in any client is difficult at best. In a CDHC, assessing motivation may be even more difficult due to the clinician's own feelings about people with HIV. If due to his or her own countertransference, a clinician feels hopeless about a client's ability to maintain sobriety because of being HIV seropositive or having AIDS, this clinician is clearly unable to do an objective evaluation and should refer the client to a colleague for a nonbiased evaluation.

It is helpful as part of the assessment process to discuss the CDHC's support network. If the CDHC has a support network which includes people with AIDS or if they had friends with HIV infection who died, this is likely to become a major treatment issue. It is important to know who in the client's support network is aware of her/his HIV infection — spouse, lover, friends, parents, siblings, landlords, employer. The client's vocational status is also an essential part of the assessment process. Is the patient disabled? If so from HIV infection, chemical dependency, or both? Often, a client desires to remain in the disabled state. This may not be in the best interest of the client's sobriety.

Though there is not yet substantive data on how detoxification may be physiologically different for CDHCs it is my observation that often the detoxification process is more complicated. Theoretically, the detoxification process, which frequently involves much stress and discomfort, can exacerbate immune suppression in an HIV positive patient.

It is essential that the medical team thoroughly evaluate a client's medical status on admission. Blood work including CBC, liver function tests, electrolytes, kidney function, and blood sugar is optimal. For the CDHC a T-Cell count should also be completed if it has not been done within the three months prior to admission. P-24 Antigen, and Beta-2 Microglobulin might also be ordered as part of the workup. HIV positive clients must also be evaluated for the possible presence of opportunistic infections. Common signs and symptoms of withdrawal from drugs such as fever or elevated pulse rate can represent other serious medical situations in someone who has AIDS. Consultation with AIDS specialists would be appropriate in the face of any symptom that might be caused by an opportunistic infection.

In a CDHC, it may be impossible to differentiate between the physical or psychiatric symptoms caused by drug use or withdrawal as opposed to organicity related to HIV infection. Therefore, it is the task of the medical team of a residential treatment center to closely monitor these clients with frequent hands-on evaluation and follow-up testing.

In summary, assessment of a CDHC must be comprehensive, thorough, and multidimensional. The goal of the assessment is to evaluate chemical dependency and those areas that have exacerbated the use of mood-altering chemicals. The second part of the assessment is describing how each part of a person's makeup affects her/his ability to maintain sobriety. When evaluating a CDHC, the effect of HIV must be taken into account as the assessment process is accomplished. Potential areas of difficulty and specific ways in which HIV is likely to impact a client's recovery must be integrated into the overall treatment planning process that evolves from the assessment.

TREATMENT PLANNING

The treatment planning process in residential treatment centers involves applying the findings of the assessment to the client's treatment stay by developing goals to (1) foster ongoing sobriety, (2) minimize complications and the likelihood of relapse, and (3) enhance the quality of the sobriety. It is well known to chemical dependency professionals that the more quality and serenity in a client's life, the more likely she/he is to stay sober.

One treatment plan centers around the goal of achieving quality sobriety. Introduction to techniques which foster long-term abstinence, such as problem solving, relating with others, and coping with stressors are included in such a plan. Other treatment plans depend on the individual's needs which might include goals about vocational or educational needs, family, relationship, treatment of depression or other psychiatric illness, and the need to deal with some issues from the past. In clients who have relapsed, specific treatment plans will focus on relapse prevention.

For CDHCs, the primary goals of treatment are the same. It is important when designing a treatment plan for a CDHC to also assess and plan for the impact of the client's HIV on their ability to remain sober. One trap that some chemical dependency professionals fall into frequently is treating a client's response to her/his HIV infection in the same way that they might treat chemical dependency. After all, both are chronic illnesses which tend to progress and if untreated eventually may be fatal.

The role of denial in a chemically dependent person may be different from that of an HIV infected person, especially if the client is asymptomatic. A CDHC may have years before she/he manifests any actual symptoms of HIV infection. It may be totally unrealistic for such a person to deal regularly in any depth with feelings of grief, fear of disability, or eventual debilitation and death.

Many clients will discuss these concerns and be able to work on them while in chemical dependency treatment. However, many others will be resistant, having successfully suppressed these emotions. The job of the professional is to assess how functional it is for the client to suppress these feelings while he or she does the early work of recovery. If deemed appropriate, such denial can be enhanced and the client reminded that he/she may need to deal with these feelings in the future through an appropriate referral source. The client is then able to concentrate on other areas of the treatment plan.

For clients who are ready to deal with their feelings about HIV infection, an appropriate plan must include balancing negative feelings with hopefulness. One of the best environments in which to do this is with other HIV infected clients. Support groups specifically for CDHCs are helpful to many of these clients whether these groups are held in the facility or in the surrounding community. It is essential for every client who is willing to participate in such groups to be able to do so as often as possible. It is important to monitor how these support groups are interfacing with the client's treatment for chemical dependency.

Part of the treatment planning process for CDHCs is deciding how they will handle their infection while they are a part of the residential community. Secrets are the enemy of recovery. However, revealing information about HIV status can be difficult and traumatic. Discrimination, fear, and rejection run rampant in many areas where someone might reveal his/her HIV status. It is the job of the treatment team to assess the safety of an environment before they encourage a client to "come out" about their HIV status. One way to do this would be to "test the waters" in a facility where there are not many cases of HIV infection. If it is not safe and the environment can not lend support to a client who is HIV positive, it is best for the client not to reveal his/her status to the community. Ideally that client should be transferred to a facility where she/he can receive support for his/her status as an HIV positive person.

A similar assessment must be made with families of CDHCs. Many families are not capable of supporting an HIV positive person in a healthy way. Disclosure to a nonsupportive family who may reject the CDHC is likely to cause such a high level of stress for the client that he or she is at risk for relapsing into use of alcohol or drugs. For such people, developing an alternative supportive family environment is necessary. This may include professionals as well as peers from a local AIDS service organization or self-help group. Staff should be prepared to work with families who are informed about a client's HIV status since such information whether or not it is new has an impact on family dynamics in recovery and needs to be addressed as part of family treatment planning. Involvement of such families in the treatment process is extremely important.

If a treatment facility contains clients or staff who are not supportive of HIV positive clients, these attitudes must be addressed by a program of client and staff education about AIDS. As increasing numbers of CDHCs are seeking residential treatment, it would be unfair as well as unethical to exclude them from treatment merely because of other clients' unfounded fears. Therefore, educational efforts organized by staff about HIV infection should be an essential part of the treatment program in any chemical dependency treatment setting. Education alone is often not enough to lesson the fear and negative attitudes many clients have about HIV infection, and staff need to work with clients on these attitudes.

CONTINUING CARE PLANNING

An important part of residential treatment is preparing clients to enter the world. Assessment of continuing care needs begins early in the process of residential treatment. The goal of the team in constructing a continuing care plan is to prevent relapse to chemical use. The first decision to be made by the treatment team is whether or not this client is likely to maintain sobriety as an outpatient after discharge. If this is not the case, then after residential treatment, the client might be better off entering longer term residential treatment or a transitional living setting (3/4 or 1/2 way house).

The cornerstone of most residential treatment centers in this country is the Twelve Steps of Alcoholics Anonymous, Narcotics Anonymous, and Cocaine Anonymous. HIV positive clients benefit from this model of recovery. Special needs of dually diagnosed clients must be considered. Are traditional Twelve-Step programs available to clients in their home area? Are those programs supportive of HIV positive people? Though "love and tolerance" is the creed of Alcoholic Anonymous, many AA groups have difficulty dealing with people who have differences such as HIV infection. Research must be done by the treatment staff as to what type of groups are available and how appropriate and supportive they would be to someone who is HIV positive. An HIV positive client is better served by a group that supports him/her as an HIV positive person than a Twelve-Step group that goes not. It is optimal to find a group that would support both needs in the client's home community. Obviously this is more likely to occur in a larger community that has other people with this dual condition. If such resources are not available, the client and the staff might consider relocation or a transitional living setting as options.

It is customary for a client to acquire a sponsor as part of 12-Step recovery. Recommendations for a sponsor who would best serve an HIV positive client should be individualized, and perhaps the utilization of 2 sponsors may be advisable; one with HIV infection (or at least knowledgeable about it) and one without.

An assessment of the client's support from family and the support that the family might need in recovery are part of continuing care planning. Many families need some extra help in the form of individual or family counseling. Support groups for families of Persons Living with AIDS (PLWA's) and referrals for counseling ought to be made available to families as part of ongoing recovery continuing care planning.

It is essential to try to ensure that clients have access to a physician who is knowledgeable and sensitive to needs of people who are both HIV positive and chemically dependent as part of the continuing care plan.

Creating opportunities and providing resources for clients who want to express their feelings about their HIV positive status is of primary importance in the continuing care of CDHCs. It is important for clients to express their feelings about their HIV positive status *when* these feelings arise. An adequate source of support for this *anticipated* need is an important relapse prevention method. Therefore, an adequate exploration of alternatives including HIV support groups, individual counseling, Twelve-Step groups, and therapy groups is crucial.

There is often guilt and shame associated with the diagnosis of HIV infection, especially for clients who have been chemically dependent. For CDHCs spirituality is as important or more important than for other chemically dependent clients. Despite the fact that many HIV positive people live long and productive lives without any signs or symptoms, often the diagnosis of HIV positivity forces people to confront their own mortality. A spiritual connection is often the cornerstone of a hopeful attitude in response to HIV. Such faith may well correlate with a better prognosis for CDHCs.

CONCLUSION

Clinicians in the chemical dependence treatment field must be prepared to treat CDHCs, and must continuously learn how to treat both the diseases of addiction and HIV infection. Those of us who already have experience in this area have an obligation to train other colleagues who have less or no experience in working with CDHCs. By serving these clients well we will enhance our own experience of recovery and survival for these clients in whom recovery "one day at a time" is truly precious.

SUGGESTED READING

HIVIES Manual, (1989). HIVIES Group, Glenview, IL.

Kain, C. (1989). *No Longer Immune: A Counselor's Guide to AIDS*, Alexandria, Va: American Association for Counseling and Development.

Pohl, M., Kay, D., and Toft, D. (1990). *The caregivers' journey: when you love someone with AIDS*, Center City, Mn.: Hazelden Educational Materials.

Ryan, C., and Pohl, M. (1990). *AIDS protocol: AIDS education and risk reduction counseling in chemical dependency treatment settings*, Rockville, MD.: Addiction Recovery Corporation Research Foundation.

Seminara, D., Watson, R., and Pawlowski, A. (1990). *Alcohol, immunomodulation, and AIDS*, New York: Alan R. Liss, Inc.

Siegel, L. (1988). *AIDS and Substance Abuse*, New York: Harrington Park Press.

Siegel, L., and Karcoch, M. (1989). *AIDS: The Drug and Alcohol Connection*, Center City, MN.: Hazelden.

Effective AIDS Prevention with Active Drug Users: The Harm Reduction Model

Edith Springer, MSW

As the face of the HIV/AIDS pandemic in the United States changes from that of a middle class white gay or bisexual male to that of a poor black or Latino heterosexual male, female or baby, it becomes increasingly clear that interventions which may have been successful in producing risk-reduction behavior change with gay men are showing scant success with active drug users. Part of the problem is our cultural assumption that drugs and drug use are intrinsically bad, unhealthy, and pathological. The general public, drug treatment workers, and other health care professionals believe this and often the drug user him- or herself has internalized this idea. People need to feel worthwhile and empowered in order to make difficult changes in their lives; starting from the perspective that what one does is bad—or that one's entire life is pathological— is a setup for failure.

Since what we're doing now is not working, it is imperative that we develop a new response to the issue of drug use, particularly in the face of HIV/AIDS. We must put our old beliefs aside and look at drug use and drug users in a new way. Only after we do this can our AIDS prevention efforts start to bear fruit. The Harm Reduction Model from Merseyside, England, is a new philosophy and strategy which has proven successful not only in Merseyside and other places in England; but in, among other places, the Netherlands, Australia, and Tacoma, Washington. It behooves those of us working in the United States to learn from the successes of others rather than to repeat the use of interventions which guarantee our failure and the consequent loss of many lives.

141

DRUGS AND DRUG USERS:
A NEW PHILOSOPHY

It may seem a revolutionary and controversial position to embrace, but the fact is that drugs are not bad. As stated by the Institute for the study of Drug Dependance:

> The vast majority of people who use drugs come to no harm, and many will feel they have benefited from the effects of drugs in improving their social, intellectual, or physical performance or helping them to relax. And they may well be right! But there are very serious risks associated with taking drugs and some of the most important points to be made about the risks of drug taking apply to all or most drugs, whether they are illegal or not. (1988)

Approximately ten percent of the people who use drugs have great difficulty with them; most of these people can be referred to as heavy or compulsive drug users or chaotic drug users. Most likely ten-percent of the population has problems with food also, either undereating, overeating, or having a compulsive food disorder. We do not, however, conclude from this that food is bad, that eating food is bad, and that people who eat food are bad. Similarly, many people enjoy the convenience of driving cars. A small percentage of these people are unsafe and chaotic drivers who place themselves and others at risk. We do not conclude that automobiles are bad and therefore should be illegal. Even so, drugs and drug use have become universally seen as evils. As health care professionals, we cannot fall prey to such moralistic and unscientific thinking. As Weil and Rosen, (1983) note:

> As long as society continues to call all those who take disapproved substances 'drug abusers,' it will have an insoluble problem of enormous proportions. Real drug abusers are those in bad relationships with drugs, whether the drugs are approved or disapproved by society. . . .

The first guideline, then, for those working with drug users is to view a drug user as a person who uses drugs, period. Drug users come in all colors, in both genders, in almost all age groups; they are poor, middle class and rich; they are gay, bisexual and straight; they are someone's mother or father, sister or brother, daughter or son, friend, lover or spouse. Drug users are us.

ARE DRUG USERS DISHONEST?

If we eliminate the "given" that drugs are bad, we can start to talk to drug users honestly and completely about their drug use. Drug use can be talked about like any other behavior that people may engage in. Then workers and clients can work together to explore strategies and alternatives. But as long as we stigmatize drug users, they will be unable to be open with us, and we set up a situation of mistrust, denial, lying, and manipulation. When working with drug users, we must acknowledge that there are benefits to drug use and they may enjoy drug use. Even when drug use is a coping mechanism that is failing to help them because their drug use has become compulsive and chaotic, we need to acknowledge that drugs had a positive meaning in their lives at one time. One of the ways clinicians can engage drug users in frank conversations about their drug use is to begin the approach on a positive note, such as, "How's the quality of the _____(fill in whatever drug they are using) out there these days?" This statement indicates that you acknowledge that clients enjoy drugs, that drugs are enjoyable, and that you have no agenda of judgment.

Many if not most of the drug using clients we see have been using drugs as a coping mechanism. Often these are the drug users who are having problem relationships with drugs. (Those in good relationships with drugs rarely come for help with drug-related problems.) A large proportion of them are compulsive, addicted, and chaotic. Let's look at who they are for a moment. The majority are poor, in fact they are an underclass characterized by homelessness; lack of education; lack of survival needs such as food, clothing, medical care, loving concern, and hope. Many are African or Caribbean Americans or Latinos who suffer from institutionalized racism and ethnocentrism which are pervasive in our country. They live often in ghettos in which their chance for success is through a separate non-mainstream economic system involving illegal activities, such as drug dealing, illegal gambling operations, prostitution, stealing, and fencing stolen goods. Their role models are those who have become powerful and prosperous in this illegal and brutal world. They have lost hope in themselves and in the American dream. In many cases, they have given up the thought of true equality and integration and increasingly accepted their disenfranchisement. A poverty of spirit is evident when you talk to them. The role of drugs in their lives is often that of a coping tool without which they might commit homicide or suicide, so great is their rage and their depression. In fact, when you look at their use of drugs, you see that it is a somewhat healthy attempt to cope and survive. For the drug users described above, drugs are not the problem. The problems are those of a deprived, stigmatized, and written off underclass. These individuals view drugs as the *only solution*. Drugs serve as a defense mechanism and coping strategy for those whose ego defenses are overwhelmed and unable to maintain psychological equilibrium. Drugs would not be a major problem for this group if drugs were decriminalized. The majority of problems drug users have with drugs have nothing to do with drug use itself but with the criminalization of drug use.

DEALING WITH DRUGS
AS A COPING MECHANISM

In psychotherapeutic training, we are taught never to remove a defense mechanism until there is another in its place; otherwise, we run the risk of causing a person to decompensate and become worse off than when he or she was before they used the regressive or harmful defense. This is no different for drug users. It is important for workers to understand that when a person has multiple problems, one of which is drug use, ripping that defense from them as the first step is inappropriate and countertherapeutic.

DRUG USE AND AIDS PREVENTION

While we have been talking about drugs and drug use up to this point, the main concern of this article is AIDS prevention. What is the relationship between these two issues? There are several relationships between drug use and HIV/AIDS.

1. TRANSMISSION THROUGH INJECTION EQUIPMENT. The first, and most obvious, is that HIV is efficiently transmitted during the sharing of drug injection paraphernalia, including syringes, needles, cookers or spoons, cottons, and water glasses — often referred to as the drug user's "works." Due to the fact that needles and syringes are made unavailable to drug users by law in eleven states in the U.S. those who are injectors in those states do not have adequate supplies and are forced to share them.

2. THE SEX-DRUG LINK
   a. EFFECT OF COCAINE ON LIBIDO. The use of cocaine in any form has effects on the libido. In early cocaine use, the libido is stimulated, resulting in more sexual activity; with frequent high dose use of cocaine, the neurochemical dopamine becomes depleted, resulting in a loss of sexual desire.
   b. SEX FOR MONEY OR DRUGS. Many users of high dose cocaine, for example crack cocaine users, begin to sell sex for crack or for money to buy crack. They are often young teenagers of both genders and various sexual orientations who enter into unprotected sexual encounters resulting in sexually transmitted diseases, including HIV infection. There is a strong link between sexually transmitted diseases, particularly those which involve genital lesions and HIV because these infections and lesions seem to facilitate HIV transmission. In New York City, syphilis cases are up approximately 600% and gonorrhea is up about 400%. The N.Y.C. Health Department attributes this rise to the crack cocaine phenomenon (Sheiner, 1990; Kerr, 1989).
   c. MOOD-ALTERING SUBSTANCES AND RISK REDUCTION. A third link between drug use and HIV is that the use of any mood-altering substance, whether it be cocaine, amphetamines, alcohol, marijuana, etc. often results in unsafe sexual activity. The effects of drugs can reduce inhibition, cloud judgment, result in memory lapses called blackouts, and lead to false feelings of safety and lack of concern about HIV. This is an important link even for those who are experimenters or occasional users.

3. IMMUNOSUPPRESSIVE QUALITIES OF SOME DRUGS. Certain drugs, primarily alcohol, cocaine, amphetamines, and inhalant nitrates (amylnitrate and butylnitrate) are believed to damage the immune system, leaving frequent users immune suppressed and possibly more likely to have HIV exposure result in HIV infection. In addition, if they do become HIV infected, HIV spectrum disease may progress faster than in those who do not have a history of immune-suppressive drug use.

4. PEDIATRIC HIV-DRUG CONNECTION. The vast majority of pediatric AIDS cases in the United States have resulted from perinatal transmission in which one or both parents is or was a needle drug user.

5. ROLE OF INJECTION ROUTES AND ADULTERATED DRUGS. The needle route of drug administration results in a hole in the skin. Since disposable syringes and needles are reused without the proper sterilization equipment available, microorganisms can enter the body where the immune system must deal with them, adding stress to this system. In addition, due to the criminalization of drug use, the drugs taken are not pure but adulterated with other substances, called "cuts," which increase the dealer's profit but which may be harmful to the immune system of the user.

Trying to deal with the drug problem and AIDS prevention in one stroke is impossible. There are some who believe that drug treatment is the solution to the AIDS problem. Unfortunately, even if treatment were available to those who need it, which it is not, about 30-50% of the patients on one methadone program in New York are still showing positive urine toxicologies for drugs, some of which are injectable (Sorrell 1990), and the dropout rates in therapeutic communities are extremely high. Drug treatment is not the solution to the AIDS problem. Unfortunately treatment is not even the solution to the drug problem, since success rates are so low. What, then is the goal of AIDS prevention work with drug users? The goal is to prevent HIV transmission from one drug user to another, from drug users to their sexual partners, and from drug users to their unborn children. The goals of drug treatment and the goals of AIDS prevention must be seen separately. Abstinence from drugs is not the goal of AIDS prevention. While abstinence from drugs may be a strategy for *some* people in avoiding HIV infection, it is not necessary for all drug users to embrace this strategy, just as some people may choose celibacy as an AIDS prevention strategy, but it isn't necessary to be celibate in order to prevent HIV infection. As a clinician working with a drug using client who has multiple problems, don't put abstinence from drugs on the top of your treatment plan unless the client truly is committed to achieving it. Doing so will alienate the client or cause the client to begin a dishonest game with you that will color all of your work.

THE HARM REDUCTION MODEL

The Harm Reduction Model, which was developed in Mersey, England during the mid 1980s as a response to HIV/AIDS and the growing harmful consequences caused by the use of prohibited drugs, posits several fundamental principles. As Newcombe and Parry (1988) state:

1. . . . HIV/AIDS prevention takes priority over prevention of drug use because it presents a greater threat to the drug user, to the public health, and to the national economy.
2. Abstinence from drugs should not be the only objective of services to drug users because it excludes a large proportion of the people who are committed to a lifestyle of long term drug use.

This is particularly important when considering the minority underclass drug users who cling to drug use as a defense against the intolerable pain engendered by their life situations and our inability as workers to provide for their survival needs, such as housing, education, employment, nutrition, medical care, and freedom from violence and abuse. Forcing people off drugs, even during long incarcerations, does not change the situation, as most drug users revert to drug use after long periods of forced abstinence.

Newcombe and Parry (1988) add that:

Abstinence should be conceptualized as the top goal in a hierarchy of harm-reduction objectives (like a series of safety nets). That is, if some people will not abstain from drug use, then the next best step is not to banish them to the black market and the drug subculture, but to minimize the harmful consequences of their drug-taking behavior, both for the individual, the community, and society as a whole.

The quality of the lives of drug users can be improved and enhanced on many levels while they still use drugs. Drug users do not have to be homeless, hungry, and unhealthy. They don't have to become infected with HIV. They don't have to have their families broken apart. It is not necessary for them to first give up drugs before we can offer them services. Many AIDS service organizations and other providers specifically exclude active drug users from their services. This is unnecessary, contraindicated, discriminatory, and unethical. There is a belief in the drug treatment world and in other places that active users cannot benefit from any intervention except treatment leading to abstinence and that those who are intoxicated are unable to participate in interventions. This is not true. The only intervention you cannot do with intoxicated people is psychotherapy. You can provide education, assistance with strategy development, risk-reduction interventions, and support, among other types of help, and drug users can certainly benefit from the provision of concrete services and other entitlement. Some agencies just use this myth of unworkability as a rationale for their refusal to work with drug users.

Newcombe and Parry (1988) also contend that:

> . . . The most effective way of getting people to minimize the harmful effects of their drug use is to provide user-friendly services which attract them into contact and empower them to change their behavior toward a suitable intermediate objective. This means services which are accessible, confidential, informal, and relevant (client-led).

In this context "user friendly" implies low entry barriers, no waiting lists, no fees for service, anonymity if requested, client-appropriate hours of service (not worker/agency appropriate hours), community based services, outreach, and nonjudgmental stances on the part of workers. The services offered must be relevant to the clients and not merely reflect worker or agency agendas, no matter how virtuous those agendas are.

THE NEEDLE EXCHANGE PROGRAM

In most countries where harm reduction is practiced, the Needle Exchange Program is the "hook" which attracts drug users into contact with health agencies. While the provision of clean injection equipment is in itself a primary HIV prevention intervention, it is also a relevant service to clients. When operationalized in a user-friendly and nonjudgmental format, needle exchange programs will attract needle using clients and bring them into contact with providers. There was a Needle Exchange Pilot Project in New York City for ten months; however Woodrow Myers, the Commissioner of Health, canceled it, taking a moralistic position about drug users facing the consequences of their behavior. There are legal needle exchange programs in many countries in Europe, in Australia, Canada, and in the United States (Tacoma, Washington; New Haven, Connecticut) and illicit programs in San Francisco (Prevention Point) and New York City (ACT UP). The most successful and effective intervention used in other countries has been legally denied in the city which has the highest number of drug-related AIDS cases in the world.

Studies from exchange programs in Europe and data from the illicit program in San Francisco called "Prevention Point" indicate that these programs are successful in reducing the amount of equipment sharing, and in some places, like Liverpool, it can be seen that HIV can be prevented by this intervention. (The Liverpool Exchange was started in 1986; there has so far never been a drug user, woman, or baby diagnosed with AIDS in Liverpool.) It also is apparent that making needles and syringes available does not increase drug use or reduce demand for drug treatment. In many places, the demand for drug treatment increases, probably because of the contact the exchange allows between active drug users and service providers (Dolan et al. 1988; Buning et al. 1989; Clark et al. 1989).

As Newcombe (1990) states:

The Mersey Region has the highest rate of drug users receiving treatment in the country, and the region also has the lowest number of drug users who are officially known to be HIV positive. The national picture is that we are seeing an increase in the rate of HIV cases overall and among drug users, but within the Mersey region, there have been no new cases of HIV infection amongst drug users for over a year now. There are limitations to the official statistics we are using for these comparisons, but the strongest interpretation must be that the local harm reduction strategy, because of its early initiation and its comprehensive nature, is contributing to this very low rate of HIV among drug users.

In "Taking Drugs Seriously," a video program about harm reduction, the HIV infection rate for drug users in Liverpool is cited as 0.1% (Parry, 1990), whereas it is about 60% in New York.

SAFER DRUG USE

While workers should stress the strategy of not sharing clean injection equipment, they must also be realists and teach injectors how to clean equipment with bleach in case there is a necessity to share works and in cases where the origin of the equipment is not clear, like works sold on the street. Workers who do not know how to clean needles should learn to do so. Numerous AIDS service organizations, including New York City's Association for Drug Abuse Prevention and Treatment, known commonly as A.D.A.P.T., can provide this instruction.

PROPER INJECTION TECHNIQUES

Syringe exchange is one intervention leading to safer drug use, but it is not the only one. Aside from using clean equipment, there is a need to teach drug users safer injection techniques so they will not suffer from abscesses, paralysis, and loss of limbs when they inject improperly. Nurses, phlebotomists, physician's assistants, and physicians can teach such techniques. Teaching safer injection techniques to those who are already injecting multiple times a day does not sanction drug use: rather, it demonstrates concern for the health of drug injectors. Clinicians should locate medical staff who are willing to teach safer injection techniques and set up appointments for their clients to see them. It is also helpful for the clinician to attend the session and show support for this intervention and be able to discuss it with the client later.

ALTERNATE WAYS OF TAKING DRUGS

Another strategy is to try to convince injectors to try other routes of drug administration. Intranasal use may be less desirable for users because it is less cost efficient than injecting. When one injects, the entire amount of the drug gets into the bloodstream, whereas "snorting" results in a loss of some of the drug. The drug effect comes on more slowly with snorting, whereas with injecting in a vein, the drug is felt almost immediately. Still, if injectors can be convinced to return to snorting, usually the way they started to use heroin or cocaine, the risk of HIV infection from sharing injecting equipment is eliminated.

A more suitable alternative for the user is smoking drugs. Smoking involves a very quick effect, similar to intravenous injection. It also can be done with little waste. Cocaine and heroin can be smoked with pipes and other equipment or mixed with tobacco or marijuana and smoked. Changing the route of drug administration from injection to smoking or snorting is a valid AIDS prevention intervention which reduces the harm caused by drug use without demanding abstinence of the individual. Clinicians themselves can encourage their drug using clients to switch to less harmful routes of administration by discussing these changes in counseling sessions and asking the client to try it and report back what the experience was like and determine if the client can make this change permanent.

DRUG MAINTENANCE

Methadone maintenance, a substitution intervention, has been used for about twenty years in the United States as the major modality of drug treatment for opiate users. It was developed by Drs.

Vincent Dole and Marie Nyswander after many failed attempts to bring opiate users into abstinence (Dole & Nyswander, 1967). The theory behind maintenance is in fact harm reduction, i.e., that it is so difficult to get long-term opiate addicts off drugs that an intervention was needed that would allow opiate dependent individuals to get on with their lives, find housing, bring their families together, study or learn vocational skills, work, and have a decent life despite opiate addiction.

Methadone, a long acting synthetic narcotic, lasts 24-36 hours and can be administered once a day. It keeps people out of the illegal opiate market and reduces other criminal behavior of users as well. It is the treatment of choice for active heroin users who become HIV symptomatic. Unfortunately in the United States, it is implemented in a highly judgmental fashion in which urines are monitored by toxicology for the use of drugs, and "privileges" are lost if toxicologies are positive; counseling is often forced upon unwilling clients, and clients sometimes have been terminated from treatment for using drugs other than methadone. Dosages have a ceiling prescribed by law, and those who supplement their dose with illicitly obtained methadone risk expulsion.

While Dole and Nyswander believed methadone maintenance was a lifelong intervention, today's programs push eventual detoxification from methadone, as the drug-free state is more highly prized than the chemotherapeutic intervention. I overheard a nurse in a methadone program saying to a methadone client who was employed, had an intact family, and had been compliant with all program rules, "When are you going to get off this shit?" as she handed him his dose of methadone. If we refer clients to methadone maintenance, we should support the modality as a valid choice for those who are using opiates and want to normalize their lives.

If it were legal, it would make sense to maintain all chaotic drug users on their drug(s) of choice while we teach them about HIV prevention and health promotion. While clinicians in the U.S. cannot administer drugs to clients, they can adopt a less judgmental attitude toward our only maintenance modality—methadone maintenance. It is surprising how many clinicians have an antimethadone/prodrug free bias. Clients pick up on this. Very few people can stop a long-time opiate addiction through drug-free modalities;

methadone maintenance needs to be acknowledged as a more realistic intervention for most of these clients.

HOW TO TALK TO DRUG USERS

When working with drug users in a counseling or educational capacity, it is important to set up an egalitarian relationship rather than a hierarchical one. Drug users often feel inadequate to hold their own with professionals. The use of first names and elimination of titles can be a helpful way to set a tone of equality. Stephan Sorrell, MD, who runs the Substance Abuse Program at Roosevelt Hospital, introduces himself to new clients as "Stephan" and insists that they not call him "Dr. Sorrell." The results are instant: a rapport, a sense of caring. Workers are not superior to clients, they are equal. Workers may have more knowledge and skills in certain areas, but clients may also have knowledge and skills that workers don't have. Workers can teach and learn, and clients can do the same.

Ask the client how he/she uses drugs. Get him/her to show you how he/she shoots up or snorts or prepares the drug for administration. A health educator in an AIDS prevention project in Harlem, New York, was teaching a group of drug users how to clean works (Tobkes, 1990). She noticed that one of the men kept touching his pants pocket with his hands. She got an idea and said to the client, "If you have your own works with you, take them out and let's clean them." The client was reluctant, but she kept encouraging him and shortly after he took out his works and started to show them to her. Before she knew it, a second drug user produced his works also. It became a real workshop with the clients learning the correct way to clean works and the worker learning little esoteric bits about works that only drug users know. Show the client that you respect this valuable information he/she is sharing with you. Make comments like "Wow, you really know a lot about this."

Secondly, try to convey to the client that you do not have any agendas of your own about the client's drug use. As mentioned previously, asking about how good the drugs are on the street is one way to convey your nonjudgmental interest. Another is simply to tell the client that you are here to help, you do not judge the client, and whether the client stays on drugs or gets off them, you will continue to work with and support the client. If you don't know a lot about drugs, ask the client to tell you, e.g., "I've never taken crack. What is it like to smoke it?"

Starting out with an agenda of abstinence will set up a parental transference/countertransference. This is always to be avoided in working with drug users. They hear a great deal of judgment and advice from parents and nondrug using collaterals; they don't need to hear this from workers.

To engage drug users, workers must provide services which give a direct, immediate benefit. Try to ascertain what they want and give them as much of it as you can as quickly as possible. Wherever possible, see drug using clients without appointments, the moment they walk in. When you cannot see them right away, but must give them an appointment to return at a later date, try to give them something on the spot as a sample of your services. An example of something useful would be a works cleaning kit, containing bottles of bleach and alcohol, cotton, and new cookers (bottle tops) with pamphlets and condoms. A cup of coffee and a donut or a piece of candy can also convey caring. If clients are hungry, try to give them food or refer them where they can get a meal. If they are ill clad for the weather, see if you can get them some warm clothes right away. Psychoanalytic-oriented blank screen nongiving stances are inappropriate with hungry, needy, homeless drug users.

Ask the client what he/she wants. Obviously, your agency's mission will indicate what services it provides; however, ask the client, "If you could have any service you want, what do you *really* want?" Validate whatever it is that the client really wants. Then tell the client what is available. Example: You work in an AIDS service organization. The client tells you he/she wants drug treatment. Ask the client what he/she really wants. The client says, "Well, I really would like to keep using drugs, but I can't take the life any more. I'm tired and I don't feel well." You respond: "Wouldn't it be wonderful if I could send you to a doctor who would give you heroin and cocaine and you wouldn't have to worry about where your supply was coming from? I wish I could. It seems to me that if you do want to enter drug treatment, you might want to try a methadone maintenance program, which is the closest thing to what you really want.'' The worker should then explain the modality of methadone maintenance and also the drug free modalities that are available so that the client may choose the kind of available treatment which best suits him/her. Tell the client the positives and the negatives of programs. Give the client time to think about it. Discuss it with the client and significant others if the client wants your help in making a collective decision with his/her loved ones.

Tell the client that until he/she does get into treatment, there is risk associated with injecting and there are several ways to reduce that risk or eliminate it. Lay out the options for the client: cleaning works or changing the route of administration. Ask the client if he/she has ever tried smoking the heroin with the crack or alone (often called "chasing the dragon"). If not, instruct the client as to how to smoke heroin (lay the heroin powder on a piece of aluminum foil. Hold a flame under the foil right under the spot where the heroin powder is. Take a straw, often a glass straw is preferred but any kind will do, and place the straw in your mouth with the other end just above the heroin power. As the flame "cooks" the heroin powder, a stream of smoke will float up. Inhale the smoke through the straw.) Ask the client to try smoking the heroin as an experiment and see if he/she gets the desired effect. If so, the client can reduce or eliminate injecting. The type of intervention you have just performed has treated the client as an equal, tried to meet the client's needs as much as is possible given the present systems, meets the agency AIDS prevention mission, and will create a strong therapeutic alliance between client and worker.

Be honest with the client about other services and agencies. If you are referring the client to an uptight or judgmental agency, prepare the client for it. I have found it helpful to coach the client on how to behave in other agencies in order to get the desired services. It is also helpful for the worker to call the other agency so that the workers there know there is another worker on the case and that someone is watching. Abuse of drug users by human service and health care workers is institutionalized in all our systems; let other workers know that you will not tolerate it. Report any abuses to the highest authorities in agencies. We must advocate for drug using clients if things are ever to change.

CONCLUSION

Everywhere I go in human service agencies I find workers angry with drug users, feeling incompetent and frustrated, and burning out as they watch drug users get HIV infected, become symptomatic, and die. People ask what are the special skills required to help drug users to change their behaviors. There are no special skills involved. Clinicians and counselors already have the basic skills needed to work with people; what is needed is a new philosophy and set of strategies which will accomplish the prevention goals we set for our work. Everywhere I go drug users tell me they won't go to human service agencies because they are treated badly and don't get their needs met. With a harm reduction stance of no judgment, user-friendly services, and meeting clients' needs, clients will come in to agencies for help.

Harm Reduction is a philosophy for a public health approach to the issues of drug use and HIV/AIDS. It is an idea whose time has come. While it has been thrust into prominence because of the AIDS epidemic, it is a rational and effective way of helping drug users have a better and healthier life which would make sense even if there were no AIDS epidemic. Drug users, like all other human beings, have the right to enjoy happy and healthy lives, despite their choice to use drugs. Health care workers, clinicians, and other professionals need to have a model which works for clients as well as for themselves and allows them to feel competent as professionals; harm reduction is that model.

REFERENCES

Buning, E., Reid, T., Hagan, H., & Pappas, L. (1989). "Needle exchange V: update on the Netherlands and the United States," *Newsletter of the International Working Group on AIDS and IV Drug Use*, Narcotic and Drug Research, Inc. 4(2), 9.

Clark, G., Downing, M. McQuie, H., Gann, D., Dietrich, R., Case, P., Haber, J., Fergusson, B. (1989). "Street based needle exchange programs: the next step in HIV prevention: prevention point." Presentation at the Fifth International Conference on AIDS, Montreal, Canada.

Dolan, K., Alldritt, L., Donoghoe, M. (1988). *Injecting equipment exchange schemes: A preliminary report on research.* London, England: Monitoring Research Group, Sociology Department, University of London, Goldsmith's College.

Dole, V. & Nyswander, M. (1967). "Heroin addiction: a metabolic disease." *Archives of Internal Medicine.* 120(1), 19-24.

Kerr, P. (1989). "Syphilis surge with crack raises fears on spread of AIDS." *The New York Times.* B1 & B5.

Institute for the Study of Drug Dependence (ISDD), (1988). *Drugs and Drug Using: A Guide for AIDS Workers.* London, England. p 1.

Newcombe, R. (1990). Guide to the BBC2 video program *Taking Drugs Seriously*, p. 9.

Newcombe, R. & Parry, A. (1988). *The Mersey Harm-Reduction Model: A Strategy for Dealing with Drug Users.* Presentation at the International Conference on Drug Policy Reform, Bethesda, Maryland.

Parry, A. (1990). *Taking Drugs Seriously*, a video program broadcast by the BBC2, written and narrated by Mr. Parry.

Sheiner, R. (1990). Remarks made at an AIDS Training at Coney Island Hospital. Mr. Sheiner is a trainer for the New York City Department of Health, AIDS Training Institute.

Sorrell, S. (1990). Personal communication.

Tobkes, C. (1990). Personal communication.

Weil, A. & Rosen, W. (1983). *Chocolate to Morphine: Understanding Mind Active Drugs.* Boston, Mass.: Houghton Mifflin. p. 2.

Countertransference in Professionals Working with Chemically Dependent Clients with HIV

Esther Chachkes, MSW
Stuart Kaufer, MSW
Sabina Primack, MSW
Evelyn Ullah, MSW

This article is written about work conducted in a large voluntary hospital located in Manhattan. Census data from 1980 indicated that the community served by this hospital has a large minority population, predominantly Hispanic, many of them recent immigrants, who live at or below the poverty line and have the attendant health problems associated with poverty (U.S. Department of Commerce, 1981).

Countertransference can be defined as the totality of the worker's experience of a patient and represents a "potentially useful tool in coming to understand the patient and furthering the objectives of the treatment" (Tansey & Burke, 1989). Classically, it can be defined as a continuation of Freud's view of countertransference of unresolved conflicts and problems aroused in the analyst that hinder his/her effectiveness in the course of work with the patient. Reich (1951) defined countertransference as "the effect of the analyst's own unconscious needs and conflict on his understanding or technique . . . the patient represents for the analyst an object of the past on to whom past feelings and wishes are projected."

In contrast to the classical definition is a totalistic approach which views countertransference as the total emotional reaction of the analyst to the patient in the treatment situation (Aronson, 1986).

However one defines countertransference, whether it be the traditional or totalistic approaches cited above, working with people with AIDS provokes a variety of reactions within the worker which can affect the quality of the client-worker interaction. Dhooper, Royse, and Tran (1987-88) completed a comprehensive survey of social workers' attitudes towards people with AIDS. They found a disturbing level of homophobia and reluctance on the part of social workers to work with this population. Clearly, these attitudes provoke a variety of reactions in all health care professionals who work with people with AIDS. In addition, Maylon and Pinka (1983) found that health care workers involved with this population are subject to high levels of stress, anxiety, and guilt.

The purpose of this article is to demonstrate, through the use of case vignettes, how social workers have been able to use countertransference to work more effectively with their patients who have AIDS and to offer this as a relevant model to others who are engaged in this very stressful work.

When health care professionals engage people with AIDS as patients who are also chemically dependent, they most often find these patients depressed, alienated, isolated, and angry, with little hope. The patients' despair and helplessness can produce a similar despair in the worker. If the patient is unwilling to stop using illicit drugs, or to obtain and use prescribed drugs when hospitalized, the worker's response may be less than positive—he or she may have difficulty accepting continued drug use even when understanding that drug use can be seen as the least of one's problems as day to day survival or impending death from illness takes priority.

The AIDS Unit at the hospital where the authors have worked consists of a number of single rooms staffed by physicians, nurses, nurses aides, social workers, nutritionist, psychiatrist, neurologist, chaplain, and unit clerks. Each of the staff chose to work with HIV/AIDS patients resulting in minimum staff turnover. Patients are often well known from previous admissions and the long and complicated nature of treatments.

The Unit attempts to maintain a nurturing environment to help patients cope with the treatment of the disease. Acceptance by staff is especially important to patients struggling with fears of rejection and abandonment. For the drug addicted patients who are often extremely needy and who suffer from feelings of isolation, anxiety, stress and depression, any hospitalization exacerbates regressive behavior, often manifested in crisis oriented outbursts that are impulsive and demanding. Close interdisciplinary collaboration enables staff to overcome feelings of helplessness when confronted by the overwhelming demands of this particular population.

The difficult behavior of the addicted patient can be modified by providing a corrective experience through clear communication and structure. Likewise, the staff can be taught to recognize the need to set limits, not to become caught up with the patients' demands, and to convey to patients their expectations that patients take some responsibility to control their impulsivity.

CASE STUDY: MARY

The case of Mary illustrates the kind of patient who is difficult to manage when she is admitted to the Unit. She is disruptive, demanding and has frequent outbursts, and does not evoke empathy when she is an in-patient. Therefore, she often needs an advocate to enable staff who become angry at her to view her as frightened and vulnerable.

Mary is a 36 year-old African-American woman with AIDS. She was raised by her father and his family from infancy after her mother left, taking with her Mary's two older siblings. Mary never knew her mother but was told that her mother was a drug addict. Her father died in 1978 of cirrhosis of the liver, and her mother died in 1975 of addiction. Mary was reunited with her siblings several years ago for a brief period but has since lost contact with them.

Mary is a former drug addict who has been drug free for the past year attending an outpatient drug treatment program three times per week. Mary is widowed and the mother of a nine month old son who is HIV-negative and presently in foster care.

Mary was married for fifteen years to an IV drug user who died of AIDS. She always worked — as did her husband — but now she is on public assistance and has had several AIDS related hospitalizations. Her clinical state is worsening.

Social Work Intervention

Mary was referred to the social workers by staff who described her as being in crisis, crying hysterically and expressing fear and concern about the welfare of her infant son. Mary was being admitted to the Intensive Care Unit but wanted to draw up guardianship papers and make a will to ensure that the baby's father and family would not get custody after she died. The staff felt helpless and angry that the social worker was unable to provide legal services immediately at the bedside. They wanted to calm Mary at all costs. Because the social worker was not immediately available, the chaplain was asked to intervene. He wrote down Mary's wishes, witnessed and signed the testimony, and assured Mary that staff would advocate on her behalf. This apparently calmed Mary. She was discharged, however, before the social worker had an opportunity to meet her.

She subsequently came to the AIDS clinic where the social worker met her and discussed the guardianship issue. At this point Mary told the social worker about her child's foster care status and a scheduled court appointment. Mary had known in the hospital that the State was the guardian and a court appointed social worker was taking care of the case. She explained that her outburst in the hospital was a result of her fear that her concerns about her child would not be taken seriously.

The social worker met with Mary numerous times over the next few months. Initially Mary presented every problem as a life threatening issue. By understanding her reactions in terms of her feelings of helplessness and inadequacy, the social worker was helped to tolerate her outbursts. Early in their work together the social worker was constantly challenged to problem solve for her. She soon found this unproductive, and she had to encourage joint problem solving and problem exploration. Asking questions such as "What is the worst that can happen to you from this problem?" enabled Mary to focus on the issue. Statements such as, "O.K., You did not create the problem but now you have to deal with it because it is affecting your life" helped Mary engage in a problem solving process. Questions such as "What would you like to do or how would you like to handle this?" provided Mary with the needed guidance to stay connected to the "here and now." Mary responded to the idea that she could take charge of her life but that some struggles would take time and effort to resolve. She began to learn to focus on taking one step at a time. Prioritizing and taking responsibility helped her cope with her life threatening illness and with maintaining sobriety. Responding to structure and limit-setting enabled Mary to explore her feelings and to begin grieving her losses. She gained a sense of hopefulness about her efforts to regain custody of her son, and she took steps toward securing his guardianship. On some occasions she did get angry and demanding and the social worker continued to handle these outbursts by eliciting the feelings that led to these expressions.

Mary and the social worker have established a therapeutic alliance. She feels secure that she will be seen at her designated time and that her requests will be explored and seriously addressed. Tasks and follow up work are carefully explained, and she knows what is expected of her and what she can expect of the social worker. Mary also knows that the social worker will advocate on her behalf. She has learned that she does not have to "demand" attention or present her needs in a histrionic manner in order to receive help.

In outpatient sessions, the social worker felt that Mary was able to use social work interventions successfully. However, this same patient behaves very differently as an inpatient on the AIDS Unit. As the team is initially responsive to all of her requests without setting limits, she loses sight of boundaries and becomes more dependent, no longer feeling in control which frightens her. As a result, she becomes demanding of the staff and at times acts aggressively toward them. The staff, well-intentioned in their efforts to help, only perpetuate the problem by not setting limits which does not help her take responsibility for her provoking behavior. Staff responds to each of her crisis calls and then becomes angry. Eventually the nurses begin to ignore her requests or reprimand her for demanding behavior. When the nurses can no longer tolerate her demands and ignore them, Mary feels rejected and abandoned.

The social worker can help the staff recognize that limit-setting has significant therapeutic gains for a patient like Mary with poor impulse control and crisis-oriented behavior. The social worker can sensitize staff to the fact that anger and frustration are reactions and responses to difficult situations and are countertransferential feelings.

On the Unit it is the social worker's legitimate role to help staff recognize that responding to all the demands of a patient and not encouraging the patient to take responsibility to control his/her behavior may produce anger and, at times, even rage despite the best intentioned efforts to provide a needy patient with responsive care. An all-encompassing need to respond does not quell but often exacerbates the impulse-ridden behavior of the addicted patient because his/her capacity to take charge is not acknowledged. Many patients feel increased dependency when hospitalized. For addicted patients like Mary, what happens on admission to the hospital is that the propensity for increased dependency fosters increased demands. Clear communication of what is acceptable behavior will help addicted patients to act appropriately and to recognize that a caring and empathic staff can not be perceived as an indulgent family to be manipulated.

In addition to management issues, staff must cope with the fear and anxiety of death and the process of dying. Helping patients cope involves responding to their multiple needs, speaking frankly to their experiences and life styles, and being aware of the emotional manifestations relevant to each aspect of the illness.

Reflecting on one's fears and prejudices regarding drug use and possible antisocial and criminal behavior will help the worker tolerate the demands and needs of such patients. For many drug addicts, sociopathic criminal behavior is often part of their life experience. Many have been in jail and have committed serious crimes. Finding a point of empathy and a way to remain connected to the patient is critical.

CASE STUDY: JOSE

Jose was admitted to the AIDS Unit with PCP and a confirmed AIDS diagnosis. He admitted to a long standing history of IV drug use and injecting himself with heroin prior to admission.

Jose is a 36 year-old Hispanic man who has been a drug addict for over 20 years. His only period of sobriety was during his five years in prison from age 19—24. After his release, he resumed IV drug use and has been unable to abstain.

During his hospitalization he claimed his primary focus was abstinence and that he wanted help mainly with follow-up resources. He was charming, quite appealing, and he appeared repentant and full of self-blame. What he was displaying was a carefully censored self.

Aware of the manipulation and Jose's difficulty in revealing his neediness, the social worker did not confront him, believing that Jose needed to be engaged first in order to address the issue of his addiction and AIDS. It became clear from discussions between Jose and the social worker that he had frequent bouts of anxiety and depression and needed hope to deal with the stress of his new illness. He was isolated and afraid of his illness, too fearful to tell his mother because of her "emotional" response. He could not disclose his diagnosis. He described their relationship as angry and confrontational, and he felt resentful that he had no other alternative and needed to return to her home. His research for housing became the symbolic search for autonomy, and he began talking about his life.

Listening to him and learning of his conflicts and humiliations helped the social worker tolerate his intensity and reframe (to herself) his manipulative behavior as stemming from his neediness and his struggles with addiction as well as issues of death and dying. For this macho man, whose life was governed by fears of loss of control, AIDS only served to heighten this problem.

Jose's struggles began early in life. As a youngster, awareness of his illegitimacy caused him to feel shame and isolation. His mother left him in the care of her parents in Puerto Rico and moved to New York. Jose's grandfather punished him by beating him and tying him to chairs and tables for many hours. Jose often felt rage and anger at his mother for her abandonment. When he finally joined his mother in New York at age thirteen, she was living with a younger companion and was unavailable to her son.

Unsupervised, feeling lost and alienated from his family, he joined a street gang and began IV drug use. He was elected leader of the gang and engaged in aggressive criminal behavior, terrorizing and assaulting people without provocation. At age nineteen, he was sentenced to jail. He had already fathered two children for whom he took no responsibility. While in prison he was drug free, completed a college education and became a skilled draftsman. After his release, he worked in a supervisory capacity but resumed using drugs and soon lost this job. Addicted again, he was back on the street engaging in violent behavior. During one of the many social work treatment sessions, he finally told the social worker the details of two rapes he had committed. He felt it was important for him to come to terms with his violent past. The social worker was horrified and unsure that she could continue to work with him, struggling to find a way to feel some continued sympathy and empathy.

The AIDS diagnosis served as a constant reminder that Jose's time was limited. This helped the social worker to respond empathically and to address his fears of death. Seeing him as much the victim as the aggressor helped in her efforts to work with him. Jose remains afraid to tell his children of his AIDS diagnosis and admits freely that the possibility of their rejection is intolerable to him. He often feels despondent and sees no future for himself. He is evasive about present relationships but admits to intermittent IV drug use. As a result of their work together, the social worker was able to see Jose not only as a criminal and an IV drug addict but as a man conflicted and in pain.

CASE STUDY: HELENA

The hysteria and anger that often greets an HIV infected substance abuser was dramatically illustrated in an incident that took place in a program for substance abusing mothers with children two years or younger. This case involved all levels of staff, including doctors, nurses, security, ward clerks, and a social worker. Reactions ranged from a rescue attempt by the social worker to the demand for an immediate eviction of the patient from the hospital by other staff. It took considerable efforts to calm everyone down in order to help a frightened woman, lashing out at a bewildered staff.

Helena is a 28 year-old, African-American, single, female who was referred to Social Services during her second trimester of pregnancy upon the medical finding of a positive urine toxicology screen for cocaine. She described herself as a "recreational user" of cocaine but agreed to participate in a special project for pregnant postpartum patients as she felt the parenting classes and social work services would be beneficial. In addition, Helena stated that enrollment in the project might be a deterrent to a child abuse/neglect report and possible foster care placement of her baby.

Initially, Helena was guarded and would not divulge any psychosocial history. Thus, it was difficult to assess family and significant other support systems. She did tell staff that she had four children who were placed in kinship foster homes and that family relationships were strained.

Medical history revealed that she had a history of multiple sexually transmitted diseases, but when approached by medical staff to discuss her sexually transmitted disease history, at-risk sexual behaviors for AIDS, and transmission of infection and AIDS to the fetus, Helena protested. She adamantly stated she had previously tested negative for the AIDS virus and that further discussion of HIV counseling and testing services was unnecessary. The fear of a possible HIV/AIDS diagnosis for herself and her baby was equated with doom and perhaps imminent death. At the time Helena was not ready to acknowledge the reality of her at-risk status.

During the third trimester of pregnancy, the social worker continued to focus treatment planning on substance abuse prevention and parenting skills in addition to education regarding safer sexual practices. Helena appeared to be receptive to this intervention as she considered the social worker to be nonthreatening, nonjudgemental, and supportive.

The birth of Helena's baby in late winter was without complications. She was discharged with her infant and continued compliance with postpartum and pediatric appointments until late spring when her attendance became sporadic and then stopped entirely. All mailgrams, telegrams, and attempted home visits were unsuccessful. Finally, after a two month absence, Helena appeared at a parenting class. She was angry and was uncommunicative with peer group members.

Following this session, Helena informed her social worker that she had an active child abuse/neglect case based on an allegation of neglect two years ago which resulted in the kinship placement of her children. As goals for foster care needed reviewing and Helena expressed the desire to have her children return home, she had to demonstrate that she was enrolled in parenting skills class. A treatment plan was devised which included a contract to monitor her urine to assure she remained drug free. For several months Helena adhered to the treatment plan until the hospitalization of her baby the following December.

Her child had been admitted to the hospital with an admitting diagnosis of asthma. However, symptoms of weight loss, enlarged lymph nodes and diarrhea ensued and further medical work up indicated the need to rule out HIV infection. Helena was approached by the outpatient medical providers to sign a consent for HIV testing of her child. Frightened and angry she refused to sign the consent. The medical providers, feeling frustrated and helpless, became enraged by her refusal and verbalized their angry feelings. She then became verbally abusive refusing further treatment of her child on that day and left the clinic. Her worst fears were now becoming a reality. A team meeting was convened to inform the social worker of the preceding day's events and to work on a plan to have Helena return to clinic with her child.

During the course of the meeting, the anger and frustration of team members was expressed. Once the team could share with each other their sense of helplessness they were able to agree on a strategy to help Helena and to approach her without hostility. Following a second session, Helena agreed to sign the informed consent. She expressed her fear that should the test prove positive her family would "blame" her for transmitting the virus to her child which would result in their abandonment and her isolation. Helena was not ready to share this diagnosis with her family. She requested and relied upon the ongoing intervention of her social worker to assist in negotiating the hospital system and working through her feeling of managing such a devastating illness. The concern for her own children's health status was not an issue for her as the children had tested negative in the past. Helena was also denying that she herself could be infected.

The child did, however, test positive for AIDS, and Helena's anger coupled with the uncertainty about the illness and treatment fostered her denial further. Feeling helpless, the social worker began to view Helena as unreachable but was determined to "save" her. As the child became acutely ill and Helena continued to reject treatment and testing for herself, staff's frustration increased.

Helena perceived this frustration as rejection and continued to relate to staff with anger. She would bypass registration at the clinic and would visit the social worker first then proceed to registration for the medical visit of her child. The social worker's overidentification with this patient sanctioned this behavior.

When the child became acutely ill, there were a number of visits to the emergency room. Helena, fearing rejection and discrimination, did not inform the E.R. Staff of her child's diagnosis. Upon return to the pediatric clinic the physicians were outraged that she did not inform E.R. providers of the AIDS diagnosis as they felt it was "her responsibility" to do so. Helena felt that they were judging her as an incompetent parent. One of the doctors angrily stated to the social worker, "You should control your patient; see she does the right thing." The social worker struggled with her own angry feelings towards the patient for her poor judgment. She also felt stymied in her working with Helena who was becoming increasingly demanding and at times even verbally abusive and extremely argumentative. The social worker also felt abandoned by the team; that the sole responsibility for the patient and her child's care was now hers. At this time, Helena was also becoming increasingly withdrawn and depressed, refusing all referrals for a mental health evaluation.

At the child's next scheduled pediatric visit, Helena became quite frustrated with the long registration lines. She vented some of her anger and became embroiled in an argument with the registration clerk who she claimed handed her the clinic chart in a demeaning way. A verbal altercation escalated, and the patient provoked a fight with the clerk. She bit a physician when he had attempted to intervene. Hospital security personnel were notified as well as Risk Management. Helena and her infant were brought to Hospital Security Headquarters, and the entire clinic staff walked off in protest. The doctor who was bitten declined to press criminal charges. He understood the fear that promoted Helena's outburst. He, and the social worker, continued to press Helena to accept psychiatric help which she finally consented to.

The staff of the Pediatric Clinic had difficulty in acknowledging their avoidance of Helena. They also could not easily confront their biases, attitudes, and feelings towards this AIDS infected child and her substance abusing mother. Their reactions served to magnify the mother's anxiety, alienation, and fears. An AIDS inservice education program was held to educate all staff about the psychological and social problems frequently encountered by AIDS patients and their families. The goal of this inservice program was to improve patient-staff communication.

The clerical staff met several times with the social worker and verbalized that they felt extremely vulnerable when patients have to wait long hours before they are seen. They were concerned that this wait could produce abusive behaviors.

The case studies cited in this article demonstrate that in order to work with this population, all members of the health care team must confront their own feelings and biases in order to foster an effective treatment relationship. At present, the majority of people with AIDS are gay, poor, from minority groups, and often have a history of I.V. drug use. Prejudice and discrimination still characterize the response of many health care providers. In addition, many people with AIDS who are also chemically dependent are convicted criminals; this further influences negative attitudes on the part of professionals. The AIDS epidemic challenges health care professionals to re-evaluate their own attitudes and through this examination provides an opportunity for professional growth and more effective assistance to persons in need of service.

REFERENCES

Aronson, M. (1986). in H. Meyers, (Ed.). *In Between Analyst and Patient.* Hillsdale, NJ, Analytic Press.

Dhooper, S., Royse, D. and Tran, T. (1987-88). "Social work practitioners attitudes towards AIDS victims." *Journal of Applied Social Science.* 12(1), 108-123.

Maylon, A. & Pinka A. (1983). "AIDS: a challenge to psychology." *The Professional Psychologist.* 7(4), 1-11.

Reich, A. (1951). "On countertransference." *International Journal of Psychoanalysis.* 32(1), 25-31.

Tansey, M. & Burke, W. (1989). "Understanding countertransference, from projective identification to empathy." Hillsdale, NJ, Analytic Press.

United States Department of Commerce, Department of the Census. (1981). Washington DC.

About the Contributors

Esther Chachkes is former director of the Social Work Department at Columbia Presbyterian Medical Center in New York City.

Iris Davis is Director of Education of the AIDS Center at St. Vincent's Hospital and Medical Center, New York City.

Barbara G. Faltz is currently the AIDS Services Coordinator of the Santa Clara County Drug Abuse Services and is on the faculty of the University of California Berkeley Extension Alcohol and Drug Studies Program as well as the University of California San Francisco School of Nursing.

Michele Fontaine is the director of the AIDS mental health project at Greenwich House Counseling Center in Manhattan.

Darrell Greene is the Clinical Supervisor of Crisis Intervention Services at Gay Men's Health Crisis in New York City.

Yvonne Harris is counseling supervisor at the St. Luke's/ Roosevelt Substance Abuse Program in Manhattan.

Stuart Kaufer is a former coordinator of the Social Work Department at Columbia Presbyterian Medical Center in New York City.

Hannah Kusterer is Clinical Director of the Friendship House Association of American Indians, San Francisco, California.

Donald McVinney is coordinator of training for Client Services at Gay Men's Health Crisis. Previously he worked as a case worker/chemical dependency counselor at AIDS Related Community Services in White Plains, N.Y.

Melvin I. Pohl is Chief of Clinical Services, PRIDE Institute, Eden Prairie, Minnesota.

Sabina Primack is a supervisor in the Social Work Department at Columbia Presbyterian Medical Center in New York City.

William Reulbach was the social worker on a comprehensive care team at Montefiore Medical Center in the Bronx, N.Y. at the time this article was written.

Ron Rowell is the Executive Director of the National Native American AIDS Prevention Center in Oakland, California, and the Chair of the Board of Directors of Friendship House Association of American Indians, San Francisco, California.

Peter S is the pseudonym for a person with AIDS, who in keeping with the traditions of Alcoholics Anonymous does not wish to break his anonymity.

Edith Springer is the Project Director of the Clinton Peer AIDS Education Coalition, an AIDS prevention program for street youth in the Times Square area of Manhattan. She is also a Supervising program development specialist at the regional AIDS education and Training Center at the University of Medicine and Dentistry in Newark, New Jersey.

Evelyn Ullah is a supervisor in the Social Work Department at Columbia Presbyterian Medical Center in New York City.

Carol Weiss is a psychiatrist specializing in chemical dependency. She is on the faculty at Cornell University Medical Center and is the Substance Abuse Coordinator for their HIV Center.

Paul Zakrewski at the time this article was written was program coordinator to the volunteer visitors program to People With AIDS at Bellevue Hospital and social worker on the prison unit at Bellevue for patients with AIDS.